My Inner Journey

527 Pounds to Running Marathons

My personal story of obesity, Gastric Bypass Surgery, and my commitment to living a healthy life from the inside out.

Anita-Nell Swanson & Edwin Holtz

My Inner Journey ©2007 by
Anita-Nell Swanson & Edwin Holtz

This book is self published by Anita-Nell Swanson.

For information contact:

Anita-Nell Swanson
My Inner Journey
10400 Overland Rd, #308
Boise, ID, 83709
http://www.anita-nell.com

First Edition (paperback) - March 2007

Library of Congress Cataloging-in-Publication Data

Swanson, Anita-Nell
My Inner Journey : 527 Pounds To Running Marathons /
Anita-Nell Swanson and Edwin Holtz

ISBN-13: 978-0-9794442-1-0
ISBN-10: 0-9794442-1-7

1. Obesity. 2. Weight Loss Surgery. 3. Running. I. Title

Publisher's note:

Every effort has been made to ensure that the information contained in this book is complete and accurate. However, neither the publisher nor the author is engaged in rendering professional advice or services to the individual reader. The ideas, procedures, and suggestions contained in this book are not intended as a substitute for consulting with your physician. All matters regarding your health require medical supervision. Neither the author nor the publisher shall be liable or responsible for any loss or damage allegedly arising from any information or suggestion in this book. The opinions expressed in this book represent the personal views of the author Anita-Nell Swanson.

Cover Design

Bruce Vanderjagt
Vanderjagt Creates
http://www.vanderjagtcreates.com

Some photos in the chapter 17 taken by:

IdahoSportsPics
Scott Rasmussen & Jim Larson
http://www.idahosportspics.com

I dedicate this book to all who have chosen to read My Inner Journey. I hope my weight loss journey will inspire you to make a lifetime change to live healthy from the inside out.

THANKS FOR BUILDING STRONG KIDS!

Special Thanks

Writing this book was quite an adventure, and very fun. But without the supporting cast of wonderful people who helped out, my weight loss journey, let alone this book, may not have been completed. With that said, I would like to offer special thanks to the following people.

Dr. Oakley: Not only for a perfect surgery, an awesome challenge, but for the great material you supplied for this book. Further comments from Dr. Oakley can be found on Anita-Nell.com. Thanks to Jennifer and the entire team for your support in the office and at our monthly meetings.

Sheryl Parks: For taking the time out of her busy schedule to help edit this book. Good luck with your weight loss journey!

Kim Stewart: Owner of Powerhouse Pilates for our early morning bike spinning, training me in kettlebells, and your help in brainstorming the title of the book (My Inner Journey).

Dana Mercado: For supporting me through the thick and thin times. You have been a true friend; thanks for your honesty.

Montel Williams, Oprah Winfrey, and Bill Phillips: If it wasn't for your shows, and guest Mr. Phillips, I may not have made the choices I made. Thank You!

Disney Pals: Thank you all for never looking at me for my size but always though my heart.
Disney Runners: Malinda, Lori, Hami, Debbie, and the Disney volunteers and great supporters, Faith, Dana, Elizabeth, Linda, and Heidi W.

My running teammates: Thanks for taking the challenge. It has been an honor running and walking with you. It's very fulfilling to see each and every one of you cross the finish line. Machelle, Linda B, Tammy, Jen, Heidi H, Carol, Amy, Colleen, Connie, Jennifer, Justine, Carrie, Donna, Steve & Mike from Boise Runwalkclub.com.

Chip Morgan: Thanks for all your help on the website and for all the valuable information on getting started. I will remember your kindness forever.

Ed Holtz: My brother and the co-author of this book. Thanks Eb for giving up your time from your family and believing in my journey enough to help me put it on paper. I can never replace the experience we have shared, I love you.

Table of Contents

Forward

Astoundingly, two of every three adults in America are overweight and one in three is "obese." Furthermore, one in every twenty Americans is severely obese…. approximately 100 pounds over their ideal body weight…just as Anita Nell was throughout much of her life....

In the midst of this societal tragedy of misinformation and despair, comes a story which Anita-Nell has been willing to share with you. Her book describes a real solution, based on scientific fact and documentation, to the problem of severe obesity. This solution has been used by over 300,000 people in this country over just the past two years, and is the product of our mainstream medical complex. Therefore, it has been tested, duplicated, challenged and verified. Surgery for weight loss--- the option Anita-Nell correctly chose--- is not a panacea and it is not perfect. It probably is not for everyone in her former situation. It is, however, even with its risks and small compromises, the only long-term solution to severe obesity known to medical science today. The statistical results are well-reported and unequivocal---but unfortunately not always as perfect as Anita-Nell has demonstrated in this wonderful story. This, then, is a sort of parable of the many permutations of what is possible with Gastric Bypass Surgery for weight loss. It is heartfelt on Anita-Nell's part, and heartwarming on our part to share this story. Not all of us can be as steadfast or as inspired as this lady is, but if this wonderful story helps to show someone in the despair of severe obesity the truth about what is possible, or gives them an avenue away from this genetically predetermined disease, then a great good has been accomplished.

Christian Oakley, M.D.

Watching Anita-Nell make significant changes in her life continues to inspire me as her coach as well as in my own personal life. Her enthusiasm and development into an athlete have been empowered by love for people as she encourages and teaches others how to make important changes in their lives. Much more than losing over 350 pounds and now running marathons, Anita-Nell's journey is all about fighting for the hearts and souls of other adults and helping them believe in themselves, helping them believe they too can go the distance, helping them believe they too can be our hero

Coach Steve Blake
BOISE RunWalk
boiserunwalk.com

Introduction

The number one question people ask me is when they find out that I have lost 365 pounds is *"Did you do it the hard way on your own, or did you take the easy way out with weight loss surgery?"*

I find this comment very offensive. I started my weight loss journey over 30 years ago, and I have tried many weight loss diets and programs, and each time I put my heart and soul into it. Somewhere along the way, I always failed and I gained the weight back. Most of the time I gained back additional weight.

I finally came to a point in my life when I realized that a diet was not the answer to losing 365 pounds. There is no magical way to lose this kind of weight. There is no easy way out.

The only way a person weighing 527 pounds is going to lose this much weight is to permanently change his or her life forever. It became crystal clear that I had to use every tool available to me. But it also meant making a personal commitment to permanent changes in the way I eat and exercise. Many people want to lose the weight, but want to do it without any type of exercise or any level of fitness. I consider this approach the easy way out, and in most cases this approach will lead to regaining some or all of the weight.

It came down to two choices for me when I weighed 527 pounds and had a Body Mass Index (BMI) of 71.1 percent. I could continue on the path of morbid obesity, and live an unhealthy life in denial, or I could choose a better quality of life and do what it takes to become healthy from the inside out. I chose the latter, and that is what this book is about.

This book will focus on my weight loss and weight gain history throughout my life. You will read about the struggles, the emotions, the eventual path that led me to Gastric Bypass Surgery at age 41, and my healthy life following my surgery.

In this book I talk about the diets, eating habits, weight loss programs, and fitness I experienced throughout my life. The most important point is that my weight problem did not just magically disappear after I had surgery. As a matter fact, that was when the hard work, dedication, and a commitment to a new life began. To become healthy from the inside out, you must commit yourself not only to surgery, but to a lifetime of nutrition, dietary supplements, and exercise. If diet and exercise alone have not worked for you, then this book is a must-read.

If you're obese, then hopefully my life story will encourage or inspire you to change your life forever too. If you're not overweight, then hopefully you will pass this book on to someone who is obese, and you will become a positive supporter in that person's life, and help them permanently change their life forever.

My weight loss journey was a long and bumpy road, and definitely was not done the easy way. I only hope after you read this book, that you will learn from my mistakes, and emulate my success, and that you too will decide to save your life, and make the necessary changes in your life to be healthy from the inside out.

Chapter 1

The Early Years

Even though a majority of my adult years were spent in a very large obese body, I actually entered this world as a smaller than normal person. I was born five weeks early as a petite, 5 pound 10 ounce baby.

Looking back at my childhood pictures, it appears I started gaining weight when I was about five years old. My weight then was considered above and beyond a normal 5-year-old child. I am one of four children. I have an older sister who is three and a half years older, and two younger brothers. One is one and a half years younger, and the baby of the family is two and a half years younger. I lived in Nashville, Tennessee during my early childhood.

I cannot pin point the exact reason why I started gaining weight, or what triggered what became a 35 year steady weight gain, but I did have trauma early on in my life which could have affected it, or maybe it did not.

Between my birth and my sister's birth, my mom miscarried one child in the first trimester of her pregnancy. So it was particularly hard the night my mom went into labor with me. The labor, all in all was easy enough, until the fifth hour when the doctor came to my mom's room and said, "The nurse is unable to find a heart beat, and we feel the baby may be dead." This was ME they were talking about. My mom became hysterical, and she was subsequently knocked out with a sedative. She only remembers waking up to a nurse saying, "Congratulations! You have a healthy baby girl!" No other explanation was given, or I guess needed at the time. Wow, childbirth in the 60's was a little bit different than it is now.

When I was three years old, my dad took all four of us kids over to our cousin's house for a backyard barbeque and summer swim. My mom was not feeling well so she stayed home. As the story goes, sometime during this outing, one of the family members said, "Hey, where's Anita-Nell?" Yep, you guessed it, I was found at the bottom of the deep end of the pool. My older cousin Becky jumped in the pool and pulled me out. CPR was not exactly the norm in the 60's, so I guess they just shook me, and pounded on my back until I finally spit up water. My personal recollection is that it was like an out-of-body experience. I could see myself being whisked into my aunt's bedroom. They laid me on her bed as I coughed up water over and over, and I remember the adults switching towels from under my chin as I coughed up the water. A little later in the day my mom was called, and my dad informed her of what had happened. When my mom asked how I was doing, my dad told her I was doing fine, and that I was lying down for a nap. That's right, a nap! No hospital, no medical follow-up, just a quick nap. That was all that was needed back when I was little girl.

My dad had several heart attacks, and he finally died of his fourth heart attack two months before my fifth birthday. His death was extremely hard on me. I was told that I could not attend his funeral. I threw an absolute fit for several days until I was finally granted permission to go. After the church services, we went to my grandma's house for an open casket viewing, and I was allowed to go up to the casket to say goodbye. Emotionally, this was probably the most traumatizing time of my early childhood.

My lifelong battle with obesity could have been physically connected with an oxygen deprivation to the brain during childbirth, or a few years later when I was found at the bottom of a swimming pool, or it could have been emotionally tied to my father's death, or maybe even a combination of all or none of the above. All I know from looking back at my childhood pictures is that my weight gain began around age five. But I was the only one who gained excessive weight. My sister and brothers did not seem to gain extra weight as I did. We all ate from the same table, and we all ate similar portions. It was not like I started eating larger portions than the rest of the family. I was definitely not a child who would ask for more; nevertheless, the weight gain began when I was around age five.

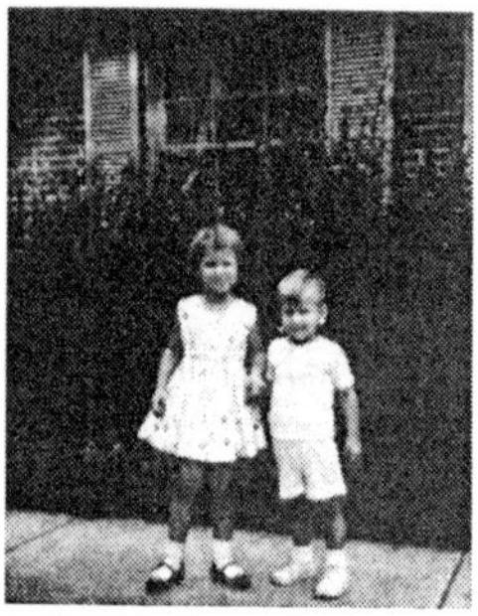

Anita-Nell, age 4, with younger brother Ed

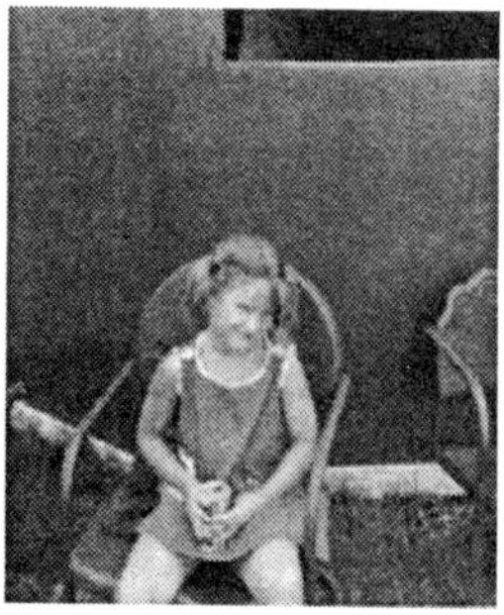

Anita-Nell, 1st grade, 6 years old

I actually remember gaining weight around the first or second grade, and being heavier than others my age. I could physically see that I was much bigger than my friends of the same age. I noticed during recess and PE that I was one of the last kids picked for a team. I was the slower runner. I did not compete as fast as the other kids. I was considered the big awkward girl to my classmates. I continued to grow bigger than normal throughout my childhood.

When I was ready to enter the third grade, my mother sold our house, packed up the family, and moved us to the Seattle area to be closer to her side of the family.

Looking back at this time period now, this was pretty traumatic as well. My dad's side of the family was all I knew. I was leaving my cousins, aunts, and uncles behind. And we were leaving my grandma (Dad's mom). She was my comfort for all my problems in life, and now we were moving 2000 miles away. My grandma was the only one who seemed to understand my problems. I was able to talk to her about anything, and she would always have the right answer for me. I was very sad that we had to move.

Chapter 2

True Friends

We moved to the Seattle area where my mom's family was living. My mom, because she was now a widow, wanted to be close to her family. I was hoping that since we were moving to be with family, that I would develop instant bonds. This was not the case at all. Even though we moved there to be close to family, it was that side of the family who began the cruelty towards me and my weight.

My most vivid memories were of my Grandma Anita-Nell, for whom I was named. She was the cruelest of all. She would come to our house over the holidays, and would ridicule me for being fat. She used to say, "You're so fat, you're not good enough to be my namesake." I remember one time that I was unloading a dishwasher, and I had trouble putting the dishes in the cupboard because I was too short, but she said, "You are tall enough to put those dishes away, but you can't because you are just too fat. That is why you cannot reach." She made many comments like that to me.

I even recall that after one of my grandmother's episodes, my aunt came to my room to comfort me as I cried. This aunt too had a weight problem when growing up. She said, "Honey, it's all right! She used to call me fat too. You may want to lose weight while you are young, it will make it a whole lot easier. That way she will have nothing to complain about later."

Looking back as an adult, and not to make excuses for my Grandma Anita-Nell's behavior, I later found out that she was an alcoholic, and was mean to most around her when she was drunk. Even though she was mean to others, I only remember the barbs she made to me. She died shortly after we moved away from the Seattle area.

My mom was the oldest of five sisters, and three of the four aunts lived in the Seattle area. Only one other aunt had kids near by when we moved to Seattle, and she had five. All were similar in age to our family. Over the three years we lived in Seattle, my five cousins ridiculed me many times over. They lived on a ranch, and used to tell me, "You are too fat to ride our horses. You will break the horse's back." There were rhymes they used to sing to hurt my feelings. My younger brothers and cousins used to sing along. "Nita Nelly big fat belly, or Nita Nell big fat bell." They would sing this over and over to hurt my feelings.

You can only go to your mom so many times about being called fat. I spent a lot of my childhood alone and crying because of this ridicule.

In Seattle, I began the new school year in the third grade. My mom contacted the school because of my size. She told me she was concerned about my weight, so she had the school nurse draw blood a few times a year to test for diabetes.

I also noticed my lunches started to change. My brothers would still get cookies or chips in their lunches; however, I would get an apple snack or a piece of fruit in my lunch instead. This was about the time I observed that my mom began to address my weight issues. She was now actively doing things differently in hopes that I would slim down.

Because I was bigger than most of the kids my age, my mom used to buy me husky clothes. Of course, the larger sizes never had the same style or look as did the normal kids' clothes. What made things even worse was that my cousins from Nashville used to send my sister their leftover clothes. But because of my size and weight, I was the recipient of the majority of these hand-me-downs. These clothes were usually the styles from many years earlier. So there I was: A little bit taller than most, quite a bit heaver than most, and definitely the worst dressed of most kids. It's amazing I ever made it through the third grade.

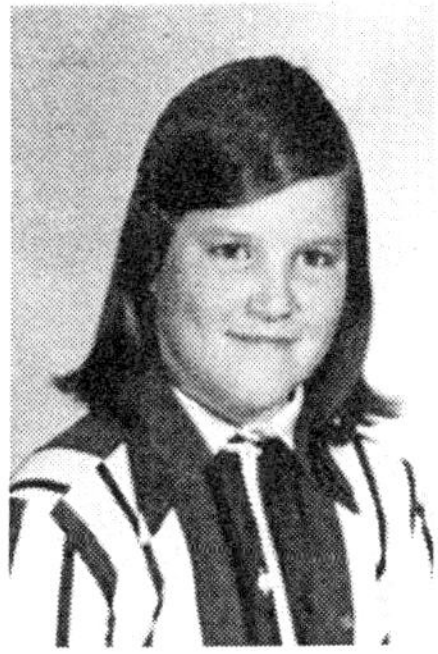

Anita-Nell, 3rd Grade, 9 years old

I recall reading a story around the time I was in the third grade about a very mean Queen who was very wealthy and large in size. She got everything she wanted. She found out about a planet made of ice cream. She so desperately wanted it, so she used her wealth to put a plan in place. She assembled a team to go and get the ice cream planet.

Once she had the planet of ice cream in tow, she realized they could not land because the ice cream planet was way too big. So while they tried to figure out how they were going to land, they just circled the earth. As they circled, the ice cream planet began to melt. It rained ice cream around the world for months. Everyone on earth was so happy. By the time the queen was finally able to land; she had lost tons of weight, and she was thin and very beautiful. She lived a long and happy life as a thin, beautiful, and nice queen.

I read this book over and over, and wished so much that I could be this beautiful, thin, and nice queen. I wished there was somewhere in space that I could go and lose my weight.

During my time in the Northwest, I did make two really good friends. Their names were Jackie and Mary Kay. They were not like most kids. They did not tease me because of my weight. No, they both accepted me for the person I was. Everything I did in life was done with either Jackie or Mary Kay.

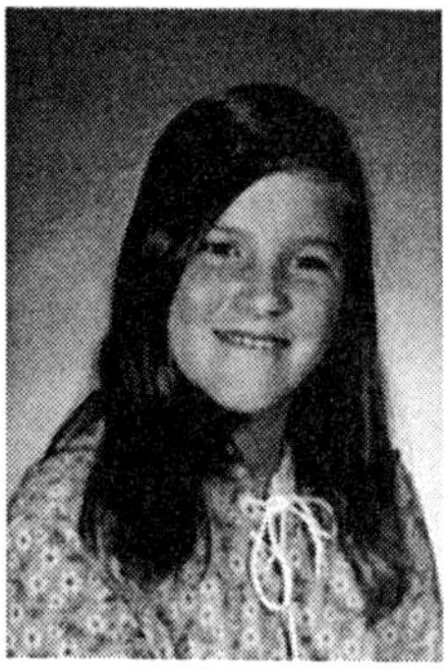

Anita-Nell, 4th grade, 10 years old

As I grew older and moved away, I kept in touch with Jackie. Jackie accepted me with unconditional love. During the three years I spent in the Northwest I spent five of the seven days a week with Jackie. We were inseparable. I sure love her; she will always be in my heart!

My mom dated a really nice man named Ron, for about four years. He lived in Northern California. She first met him in Nashville when he was visiting his sister, who happened to be my mom's best friend. They continued to date when we moved to the Northwest. He was a traveling salesman, so they would see each other when he came to the Northwest on sales calls. After three years in the Northwest, my mom and Ron got married, and they moved the family to Northern California.

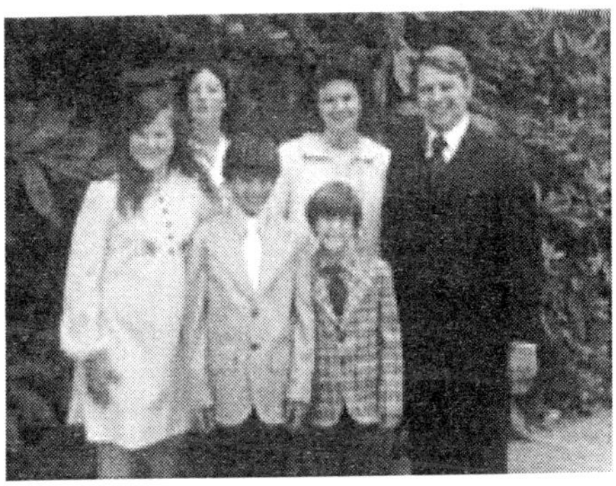

Mom and Ron's (Dad's) Wedding Day

Chapter 3

Time for Fat Camp

Yet again, I had more traumatic events in my life. I was moving away from my best friend, a grown man was now moving into our house, and once again I was going to start a new school year in a strange place.

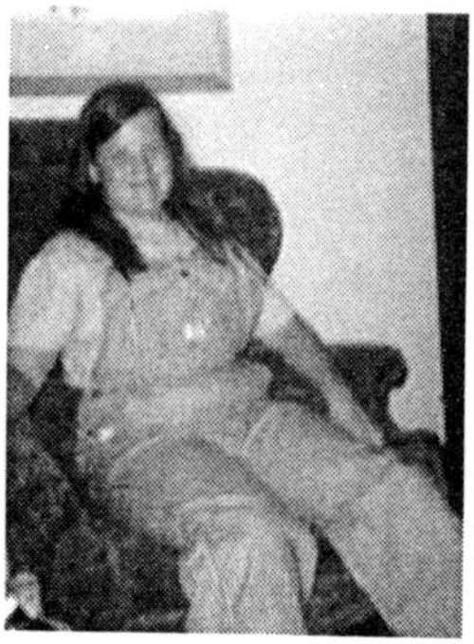

Age 12 at our new house in California

We arrived in California in the summer of 1973. I was 12 years old. California was considered, by the rest of the country, to be fast paced, and to be more modern. The only difference I noticed was that we moved into a brand-new house. We had never lived in a house that had just been built. Everything had that new smell to it. The paint, the carpets, and the vinyl flooring all released that new chemical scent and it gave me a headache.

I spent the next year making new friends, and adjusting to my new school. Shortly after we moved to California, I was thumbing through my mom's brand new subscription to Sunset Magazine, and I found an ad in the back for a Weight Watchers Camp in Southern California. I promptly asked my mom if she would pay to send me there, and the answer came back immediately that she and my new dad just did not have the money to send me. I clipped the ad anyway, and asked them on a regular basis throughout the school year. I was like the little girl who asked for a pony every day; but in my case it was a weight loss camp.

My dad did leave a decent amount of life insurance money in a Trust. After a few conversations with the trustee of the trust, my mom was able to get permission to use trust money for the Weight Watchers Camp. The trust was worded, "*For the Health, Education and Welfare of the Children,*" so the trustee agreed that my weight had become a health issue. Therefore, the cost of the camp would be covered by the trust.

I was approved to go during the summer after I finished the 6th grade. As the summer drew near, my mom took me shopping for clothes to take to camp. She took me to K-Mart. I was really embarrassed. She made me feel so fat. She bought some Blue Light Special XL polyester old lady shorts. She said, "These will have to do because you will not fit in the normal nylon shorts." Because these were on sale, she bought me eight pair of shorts in all different colors. They were horrible.

My mom drove me down to Claremont in Southern California for the first day of orientation. I weighed 196 pounds. We met with camp weight loss counselors upon arrival, and it was determined that I should set my weight loss goal at 58 pounds. My goal weight would be 138 pounds.

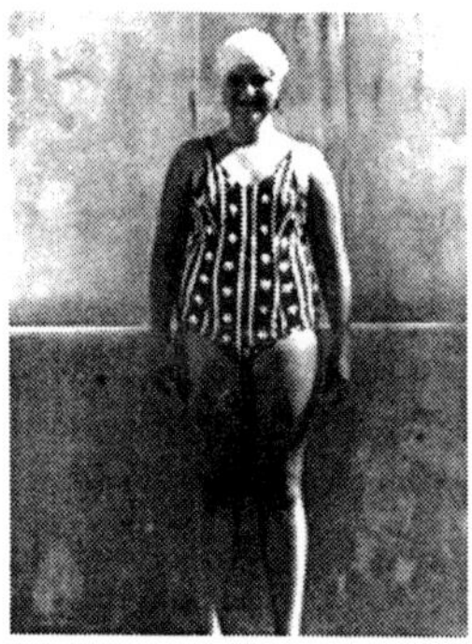

Age 13, my before picture to Weight Watcher's Camp

The camp was on a college campus with a swimming pool, tennis and basketball courts, and several fields which we used for our outdoor activities. Our dorms were set up with two campers per room, and six campers per counselor. All of our rooms were in a row in one section of the dorm.

Activities included basketball, volleyball, tennis, golf, aerobic exercise, and archery. We also had several large rooms set up for arts and crafts. Every morning before breakfast, we did 20 minutes of stretching and calisthenics. We then had one physical activity, and one quiet activity. The quiet activity would involve some kind of art or craft project, which was determined on a daily basis. Then we would do pre-lunch exercises where we worked out pretty hard for an hour. We then went to lunch.

After lunch we were given one hour of free time, and then we had two physical activities and one quiet activity. Dinner followed the afternoon activities. After dinner, the entire camp would get together and do skits, tell campfire stories, or participate in a sing-a-long. Like:

They say the boys at Claremont
Are mighty, mighty fine,
But the one across the table
Looks like Frankenstein,
Oh, gee, Mom I want to go,
Oh, gee, Mom I want to go hooommme!

The camp was seven weeks long. We were able to go on field trips to Disneyland, the Beach for the 4th of July and fireworks, Hearst Castle and Solvang (a little Danish town). Because the camp was in Southern California, there was also a chance of a celebrity sighting, and on visitation day, I did get to meet a famous actor.

I fell short of my goal weight of 138 pounds; however, I did manage to lose 41 pounds over the seven week camp. I took the train home from Southern California, and I was met by my mom.

My step dad was Catholic, so he and Mom decided over the summer to put the three youngest kids in a parochial school. So instead of following my friends to public junior high, I started the seventh grade at St. Williams.

I held my weight throughout the seventh grade, and by the end of the school year, I had only gained six pounds. At 161 pounds, my mom let me return for a second year at Weight Watchers Camp. My goal weight was the same as the year before.

This time the camp was in San Luis Obispo in Southern California. The camp was set up the same except now the dorms were upstairs and downstairs with the counselors in the dorm with the group.

This year I tried to have another star sighting, but; I did not get to meet the famous dad, Brian Wilson, from the Beach Boys, although we all did look around his limousine to try and see in. His daughter, Carnie, and nephew, Jonah Wilson, both attended the camp. Jonah ended up being my buddy. We hung out together throughout the seven week camp. Carnie Wilson, as you may well know, ended up being the poster girl for Gastric Bypass when she had her surgery in 1999.

This camp was much more enjoyable for me because I knew what to expect. At the end of camp, I reached my goal weight of 138 pounds; I had lost a total of 23 pounds.

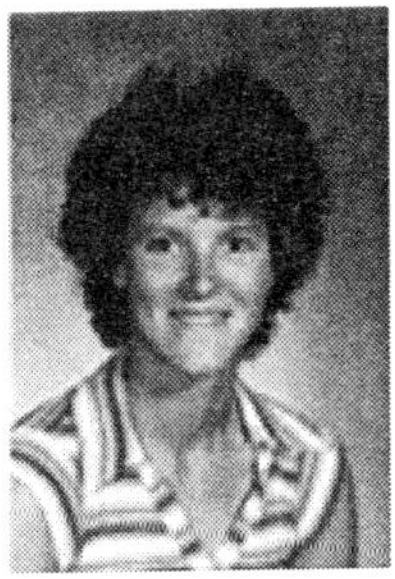

Age 16, after 2nd Weight Watchers Camp

I went to St. Williams through the eighth grade, and then returned to public high school. By the end of my sophomore year, I weighed approximately 200 pounds. I did not want to be fat anymore, so I observed my sister Johnnie and her dietary behaviors. She was skinny as a rail.

My sister Johnnie, who had recently returned from college, and who moved out on her own, became my mentor regarding food. I visited her quite often. Unconsciously, she taught me how to binge eat, and then use laxatives. She also taught me the art of starvation. I believe I went through my senior year of high school 80 percent bulimic, and 20 percent anorexic. My behavior was so bad during my senior year that I remember going 30 days only chewing sugar free gum and diet soda. I did this more than once through the year.

About midway through my senior year, I got a job at a local fast food restaurant. It was there that I met my first real boyfriend, Doug. To look good, I spent a lot of time starving myself. By the end of my senior year I had lost a total of 60 pounds, and I weighed around 140 pounds. I was now six feet tall.

Chapter 4

A Beautiful Baby Girl

I was able to maintain my weight at 140 pounds through starvation and laxatives, but by the end of my senior year, I became pregnant with my daughter.

Once I found out I was pregnant, I began to eat again. I stopped taking laxatives, and tried to get the proper nutrition for my baby. I also broke up with my daughter's father, who at the time was not interested in being a dad. He said, "The only reason you want this child is because you're just looking for a plaything." When my daughter was nine months old, I made a trip to see him, and he still was not interested; he did not even want to meet her. I inject this into the book, just so you know that I was a single mom until my daughter was 10.

I gained about 95 pounds throughout my pregnancy, and after my daughter was born, I weighed 235 pounds. When my daughter was a few months old, I once again tried the starvation, binge eating, and laxatives. However, it just wasn't the same, so after a couple of months, I quit this lifestyle of starvation and binge eating for good. This led to more eating, and I continued to gain weight until my daughter was a year old. About this time, I was tipping the scales at 270 pounds. Even at 270 pounds, I did meet a special guy at work, and I began dating him about a year later. His name was Dale, and we would date on and off for the next 10 years.

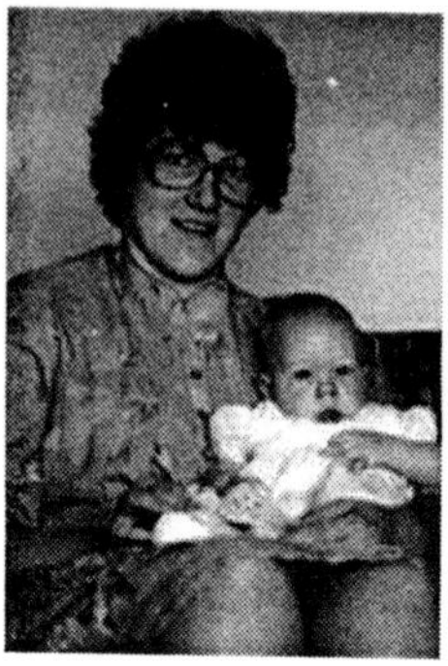

My daughter and I.

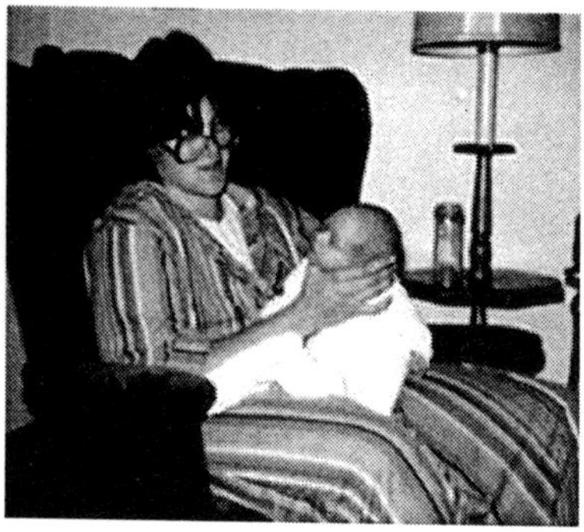

My weight was 235 pounds plus.

Emotionally I was a wreck. I let my weight go from 140 pounds to 270 pounds in just under two years. This was my biggest weight gain ever. In this short time period I had gained 130 pounds, so I decided to go back to a weight loss program. I elected to use the familiar Weight Watchers program.

I stayed on Weight Watchers for about nine months, and I was able to get down to 190 pounds. I was pretty proud of myself, I had lost 60 pounds. Just before my daughter turned two years old, I went off the Weight Watchers program, and I was able to stay level for a few months.

Sure enough, when you do not exercise or monitor your food intake, or portion size, you begin to put on the pounds. Over the next year and half I slowly put on one to three pounds a week. So when my daughter was three and a half, I was around 330 pounds. I had gained 140 pounds.

Once more, I went back on Weight Watchers for the next 18 months, and by the time my daughter was five I had returned to the familiar 200 pounds. I had lost 130 pounds on the Weight Watchers program. I stayed level for a few months, and then began to gain.

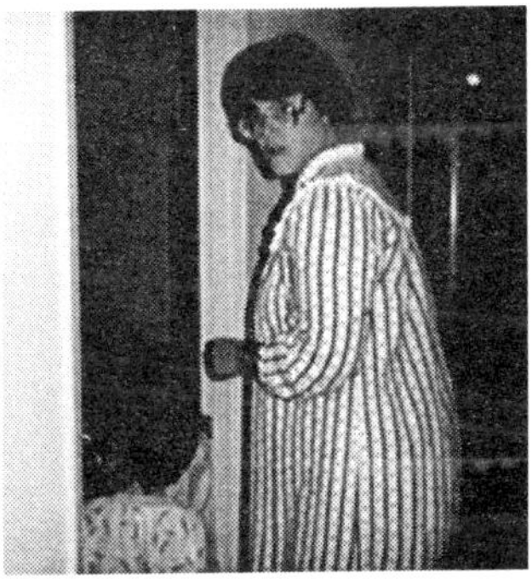

Down to 200 lbs.

Over the next year I gained back everything I had lost plus 50 more pounds. I stayed at 380 pounds for about a year. When my daughter reached age seven, I got a call from my mom. She had heard about a new weight loss program, and felt I should give it a try. It was called NutriSystems. This was in the infancy of the NutriSystems program, and only Hollywood stars and the rich were taking advantage of it. This was prior to the current $300.00 internet program. It was far from this cost.

At that time, the program was structured by how much weight you had to lose, and the length of time needed to lose that weight. My cost was going to be $1,800 plus the cost of weekly food maintenance.

My mom was extremely worried about my health, and the toll my body fat was taking on my heart, so she encouraged me to join. She agreed to pay the initial $1,800 fee, and I would pay for my weekly food.

NutriSystems was a radical change from Weight Watchers. The food and portions were pre-packaged, so there was no measuring, like there was on Weight Watchers. This was very convenient for people on the go. It was also great for me because I was a single mom who worked full time. At the time, the program seemed very high tech and upbeat. My weight loss counselor had a lot of energy, and was a great cheerleader. Everything was new and great for the first year, but after you experienced everything on their menu, it became quite bland. However, I was losing weight and it was very convenient, so I stuck with it. It took two years and a little starvation at the end, but I reached my goal of 160 pounds right before my daughter turned nine years old. Yeah! I was skinny again!

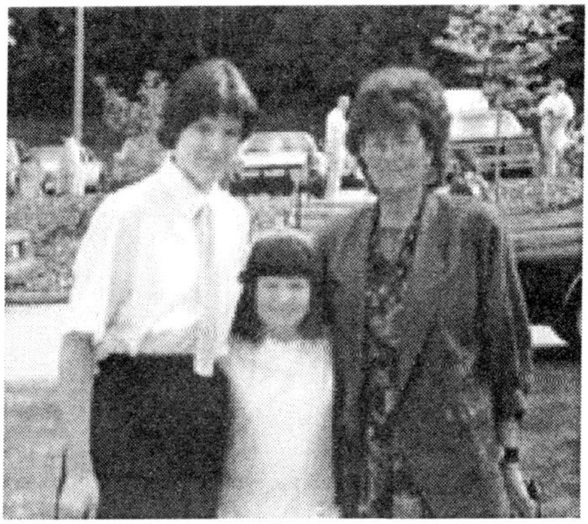

Myself, my daughter Leah, and my Aunt Judy
Spring 1989 – 160 pounds.

Chapter 5

Time to Move Again

Shortly I reached my goal weight of 160 pounds. I began to have abdominal pain. As the pain got worse, I decided to go to the emergency room. Since I was running a fever, the doctor diagnosed my pain as the flu, and sent me home.

For the six months, I would get bouts of abdominal pain, but would dismiss it as really bad gas. Then late one night the pain was so bad, I hit the floor. My daughter thought I was going to die as I rolled around on the floor in pain. She called a family friend, Julie, to come over and help out. Julie took me and my daughter to the emergency room. I was diagnosed with excessive gallstones and would need surgery to remove my gallbladder. Since I was at the hospital over the 4th of July holiday, and there was no surgeon at the hospital to do the surgery, I was sent home. I was given some pain medication and told to make an appointment the following week with a surgeon. I never made that appointment. On the following night, I again experienced extreme pain.

This time Leah, my daughter, called her grandmother for help. My mom came over and took me to the hospital. The physicians determined that I would be operated on first thing in the morning as an emergency open cholecystectomy. This meant they were going to remove my gallbladder by open surgery. They wanted me to stop any intake of food or fluid to prepare my system for surgery. My mom made arrangements for Leah to stay with other family members while I was in the hospital.

The surgeon who examined me said that the excessive build up of gallstones and malfunction of my gallbladder was caused by my recent weight loss. He said because my weight loss was not medically supervised, and because the weight loss was so rapid, that it caused my gallbladder to malfunction and fail.

However, my surgeon was very impressed that I was so committed to losing 220 pounds, so prior to my surgery; he offered to remove some of the loose skin around my abdominal region. He was not a cosmetic surgeon, but as he said, "It is a shame to have all that loose skin after such a great weight loss accomplishment." He considered the excess skin removal a bonus for a job well done.

I awoke from my surgery feeling relatively okay for just having major open surgery.

I had two drainage tubes in each side of my stomach to drain any excess fluid around the abdominal area. Over a 24 hour period no one caught that I was losing blood through those drainage tubes, and late the next day my mother says that my skin color turned whitish blue and my eyes began to sink into my skull. My mom realized something was wrong, and called for the nurse and doctor. They later discovered I lost approximately four pints of blood, or about 50 percent of my blood through those drainage tubes. Needless to say, I was rushed to the operating room for an emergency blood transfusion and another open surgery to locate and stop the internal bleeding. Thanks, Mom, for your watchful eye, concern, and mother's intuition. You saved my life!

I retuned home from the hospital at about 150 pounds, a little skinnier than when I entered. I pretty much leveled out over the next year to right around 160 pounds. I was very proud of myself. I spent that year replacing all of my clothes. Going clothes shopping was very exiting for me. I was now able to wear the clothes that I had only dreamed about. I loved to go and buy new outfits.

When my daughter was 10, the magical dream of being skinny slowly went way. I gained between three and eight pounds a month over the next year. Right before my daughter turned 11, I married that great guy that I had met at work. We had now been dating 10 years. When Dale and I married, I weighed 210 pounds.

Right about the time I got married, the company I worked for went into a tailspin for a two-year period. During this time, I did not know from day to day if I still had a job. I was in middle management, so I was not only worried about myself, but the people who I led below me. It was a stressful time, and I began emotional eating. Food was my comfort zone, so I ate. By the time my daughter had her 13th birthday, I had once again gained a majority of my weight back. I was now 350 pounds. However, it does not end here. No, I just piled more stress on my life, and continued eating.

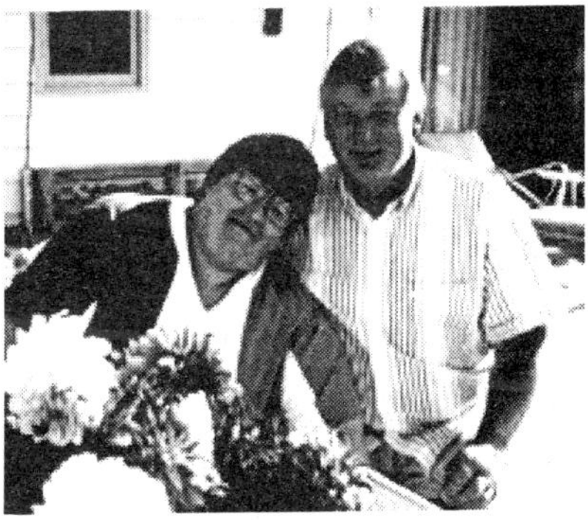

Dale and I in 1995 – My weight was now 350 pounds.

This was about time my husband had to go to Boise, Idaho on business. He returned from his trip with a new vision. He wanted to move the family to Boise. After a lot of discussions about our future and goals, we decided that we would sell our house in the Seattle area and move in with my mom for about a year while we paid down some debt. Then we would both put in for a transfer and move to Idaho.

It took about six months to sell our house, which was a little longer than we expected. After the house sold we moved into my mom's house. I had mentioned to my supervisor that Dale and I would be interested in making a lateral move and transferring to Boise as a team. About 6 weeks later, my supervisor called me into his office on Thursday, and said, "We would like you to be in Idaho on Monday if you want the job." We basically had one day to answer. Dale and I decided that I would go ahead and make the move, and Dale would stay behind until my daughter finished the rest of the school year. Our company agreed to those terms and said they would transfer Dale at that time.

The first time I saw Idaho was with suitcase in hand. For the first three weeks, I lived out of a suitcase and hotel. Dale and Leah came for Thanksgiving, and we looked at houses to buy, but ended up renting a two bedroom apartment.

I moved into the apartment by the second week of December. Dale and I flew back and forth to visit. Leah came out over her school breaks and stayed with me.
We finally found a really nice house in the suburbs of Boise, and it was priced just right. So in April of 1996 we made an offer, and it was accepted. We now owned a house in Idaho. However, I was the only one who moved in until the rest of the family joined me in June when school got out.

From November 1995 to June of 1996 I lived in Boise by myself. I tend to eat out of convenience, so I ate a lot of pizza, fast food, and of course ice cream. The weight poured on. By the end of 1996, I had gained 140 pounds.

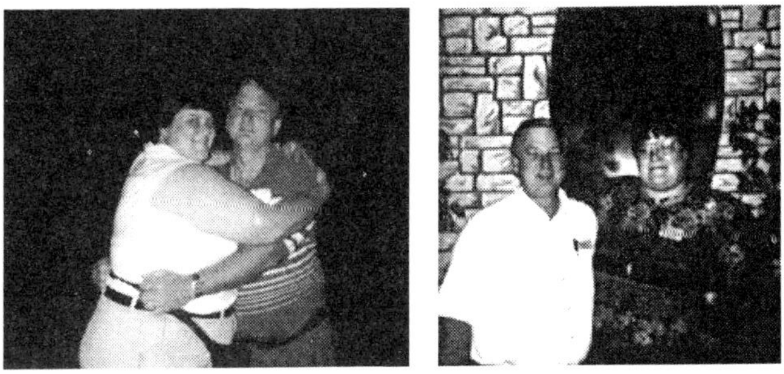

Dale and I in 1996 – 475 plus pounds.

Because of my weight, I did personally worry about my job. I thought to myself quite often: "*What if I lost my current job? Would I be employable to another company at my current size? Even though I have been with my company for 20 years, is my weight becoming a factor for continued employment?*"

Because of these thoughts, I would strive for perfection in my job. I feared that I might lose my job because of my weight, so I just worked hard at being the best that I could be. As it turned out, I found out I was considered one of the top managers in my region, so weight never became an issue.

Chapter 6

I Decided To Fight For My Life!

One day at work I began to feel chest pains. Scared, I made an appointment with the cardiologist the next day. At my appointment, I was interviewed by a cardiologist, and he wanted to run some tests, including taking pictures of my heart. However, my weight, which was still tittering around 500 pounds, exceeded the capacity weight of the test machine. I was too fat to take the test. At first he was going to set up a test out of state, but later found a local hospital that could accommodate my size.

He could not do the traditional stress test either, because I was also too heavy for the treadmill, and he did not feel I would be able to handle that test. So they ended up giving me some kind shot that made my heart race for 20 minutes. I never felt my heart beat as fast as it was beating during this test. Even up to the present day, I have never felt my heart beating that fast. I thought it was going to pound out of my chest.

After getting the second test done, the cardiologist determined the pain was not a heart attack, but was stress induced, and I was given one of those no-brainer diagnoses. Take it easy, and lose some weight. He had me take an aspirin daily, and carry nitroglycerin just in case. I did this for two years.

He felt I was one of those walking heart attacks just waiting to happen.

Within a month of my chest pains, I started having vaginal bleeding and blood clots. I did see a doctor concerning this, but this doctor just associated it with my weight and menstrual cycle. Up until that time, it had been nothing more than spotty. Over a 13-month period it got progressively worse, to the point where Dale had to wake me up during the middle of the night to change the towel on our bed. By the last month I was going through two boxes of pads and one box of tampons a week. I started having accidents more frequently out of the house, which would require me to go home, shower, and change my blood-stained clothes.

I finally switched doctors, and was properly tested. I was diagnosed as anemic. This doctor decided I needed a hysterectomy. I had the hysterectomy surgery a week later, and the bleeding stopped. I came home from the hospital at a slender 490 pounds.

During this time period, it finally hit me. I could not fool myself any longer with the patented line, "I feel very happy and comfortable at this weight." It was time for a change in thinking. I felt that if I did nothing about my health, I would most likely end up bed ridden. So it was time for me to FIGHT FOR MY LIFE!

So with many conversations with my husband about my health, we both decided to go on a low-fat diet, and started a walking program. Dale is a very supportive man (That's one of the reasons I married him). He was very supportive in my life then, and is very much so now.

I remember the first time we went outside to walk. I could barely make it around the block. I almost passed out. However, every time we went walking, it got a little easier and we were able to go a little further until we were walking about a mile a night.

Over the next few months, I did start to lose weight. I was able to shed 40 pounds. I was down to 450 pounds, and I had lost a few dress sizes.

Later that summer, my eldest stepdaughter, Kristen, from Dale's first marriage, came to visit us in Idaho. After a couple of days with us, she became very concerned about our high carbohydrate intake. Not that she was a dietitian or anything, but she did notice that we were eating a lot of carbs.

Once Kristen returned home, she did some research and emailed us the name of the latest diet that had a lot of press. It was called, *Eat Right for Your Blood Type.*

So Dale and I went shopping. We bought *Eat Right for Your Blood Type,* and we also bought a treadmill. We wanted to make sure my weight was not going to break it, so we spent a little extra money, and got the deluxe model with an extended warranty. Dale and I knew it would be cold soon, and if we were going to continue to walk, we would have to do it inside, not outside in the snow or ice.

We both went on the diet, but because we were both different blood types, it required that we eat substantially different foods. This diet did make us feel better than the way we felt on the low fat diet. However, it was kind of a hassle, because we had to prepare two different kinds of foods for each meal. We stayed on the diet a few months and through the holidays. But we only lost a few token pounds, so we eventually gave up on it.

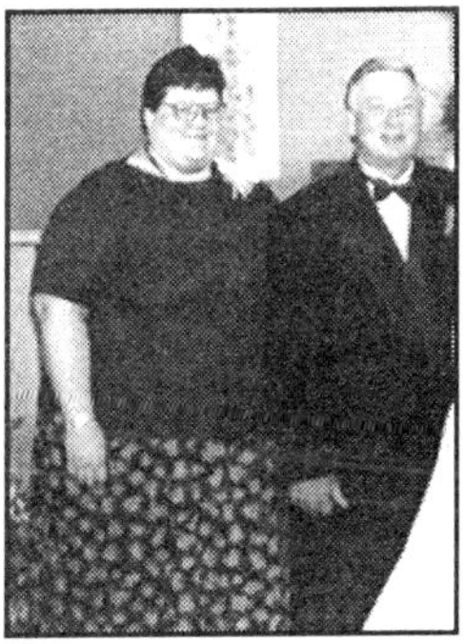

1997, Dale and I at his daughter Kristen's wedding.
I was about 450 pounds.

At this time in my life I was an emotional wreck regarding my weight. I could not even roll over on my own. I had to use the bar on the treadmill next to our bed to get out of the bed.

I remember asking Dale at the time, "So how do you like being married to a whale?" His answer was that he loved me for who I was inside, and not for my weight or physical size. You have to love that kind of man!

For the next year, I went up and down in weight, but finally topped out at 527 pounds in 1998. This was my top weight from when I actually weighed. I could have gone higher than this weight, but since I did not have a scale to weigh myself daily, this was my highest recorded weight.

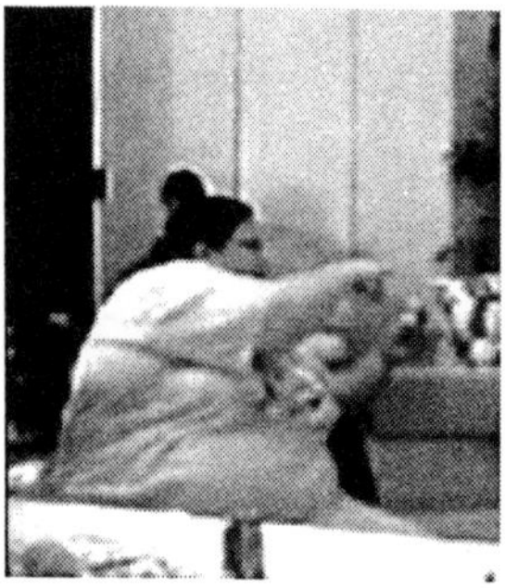

1998, my heaviest recorded weight of 527 pounds.

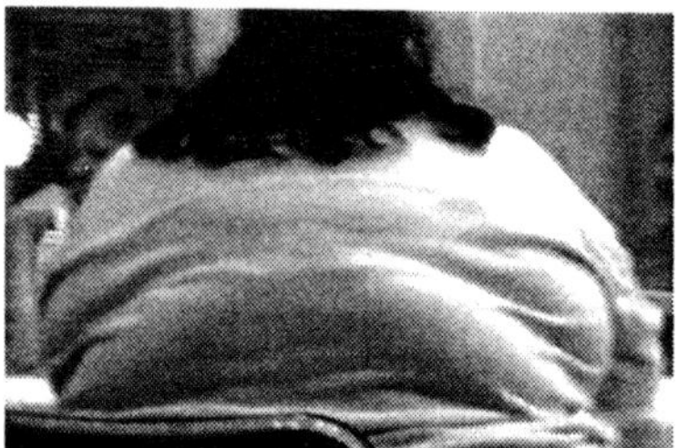

What 527 pounds looks like from behind.

To get weighed at my size, I had to go to the Post Office to use their scales, or find a hospital that had an obesity scale. Most normal scales, at that time, only went to 300 pounds.

I spent the next year telling family and friends that I was happy at this weight. I said it so often; that I actually started believing this was true. I yo-yoed up and down with my weight through the end of 1999.

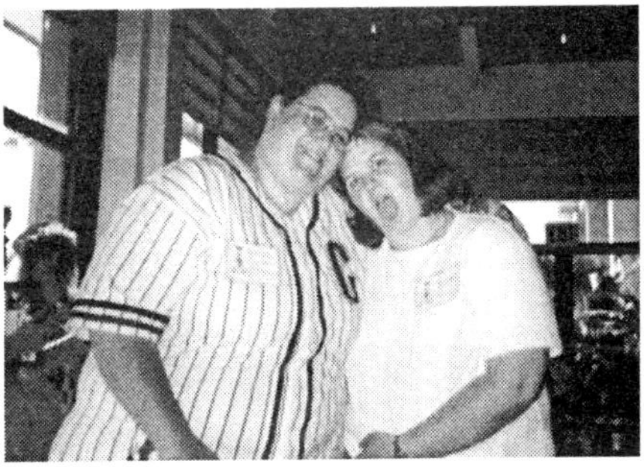

With my daughter Leah 1999.

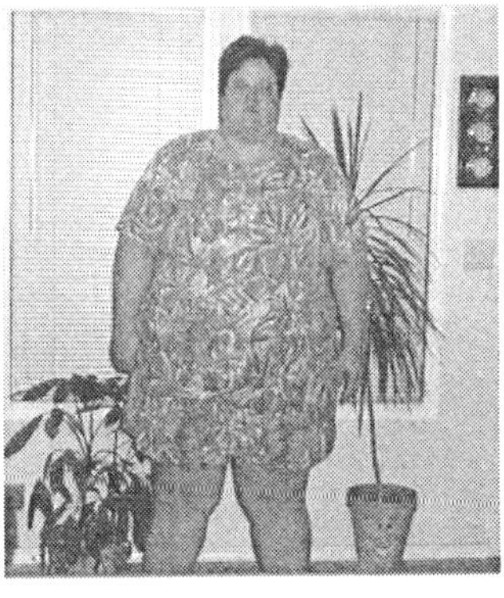

1999 around 450 pounds.

I know up until now, I have not talked about my beliefs, but I do pray a lot to God. I pray for forgiveness, for other people, for my work, for difficult situations, but on this occasion it was for an answer to my severe obesity. I begged God to hear my prayers.

Chapter 7

A Really Freaky Thing: My Prayers Were Answered Through Montel and Oprah

Okay, follow me on this one; it really was kind of freaky or weird how this happened, and looking back, it was probably the answer to my prayers.

One day I was home early from work. Okay, to be exact; it was on Wednesday, October 20, 1999. I had an all day meeting that day, but it got out early. I really did not have time left in the day to go back to work and do anything productive, so I went home early. I usually get split days off. I get one day off during the week, which I use to clean house, catch up on the laundry, grocery shop, and run errands. Then the second day off on Sunday, I generally use this day to spend time with Dale. So for the most part, I never really have the time to see any of the daytime TV shows during the week, because I don't normally get home before 7 p.m.

But this day was different. I got out of a meeting two hours early, which almost never happens. I came home, and I turned on the TV. I flipped through the channels, and I came across the Montel Williams Show. He had on a couple with before and after pictures from a weight loss program. This caught my eye. The next thing you know I was glued to the TV. The couple had just won a new Corvette, from a program called *Body for Life*. Bill

Phillips, the author of the book *Body for Life* had a 12 week challenge, and apparently this couple had won that challenge. I was totally fascinated. Not only by the prize that they won, but by the way they looked in their before and after pictures. I could not believe how well they looked in just 12 weeks. The show continued with more winners and their before and after pictures. I was totally in amazement. So I decided to write down the name of the book and its author. At the end of the show Montel made a challenge for his studio audience and the at-home audience. I was absolutely on the edge of my seat. I said to myself, *"I am doing this challenge!"*

Okay, that was easy enough and not too weird. But let me continue. What I did not know at the time was that Dale, who had been on a business trip at the same time, also had time to kill in the hotel. He flipped through the channels, and he too found the same Montel Williams Show. He also wrote down the information from the show and ordered a copy of the book. Within a couple of days, I had purchased a copy of the book locally. So a week later, neither one of was aware that the other had seen the show, or that we each had a copy of the book, and that we were both reading it.

Okay, that is a little freaky, but it gets better. A couple of weeks later, the similar scenario happened. I was at home on a day that was not my usual day off, and Dale had come home early from work. Please let me stress I never really get to watch daytime TV. However I decided once again to see what was on, and flipped through the channels. This time I stopped on the Oprah Show.

Oprah was interviewing Bill Phillips who was the author of *Body for Life* from the Montel Williams Show. This was the book that I was now reading. We both decided to sit and watch.

As you know, I had been praying for an answer to my weight in my prayers. As I watched this Oprah Show, I knew this was the definitive answer to my prayers. I was so excited. I watched and listened with great intent. I got goose bumps on my arms. I felt that this Oprah Show and the Montel Show a couple of weeks earlier were a definite message from God. How could I be so blind? The answer from God is right here in front of me.

We began to talk about the author and *Body for Life*, and that is when I found out that Dale had also seen the Montel Williams Show a couple of weeks earlier, and he too had purchased and started reading *Body for Life*. Now the hair was not only standing up on my arms, but was standing up on the back of my neck. I had a chill go up and down my spine.

We decided to follow the program together. We bought a disposable camera and took our before pictures. We went to Play-It-Again-Sports and purchased a weight set and bench. I started the challenge at 451 pounds.

We followed the book to the letter, and we had great success. We both started to lose a lot of weight.

I would always get up a couple of hours before work to do my workout with the weights. One morning I was doing "dead lifts" as part of my workout, and my back went completely out. I yelled for Dale. He came running, but could not help because the pain was so intense. Every time he would try and move me, I would scream with intense pain. So he called 911. He told the 911 operator that I was hurt, I could not move, and I was really heavy.

Two fire engines and an ambulance arrived at our house with their sirens on at 6:00 a.m. Eight fighters and paramedics entered my living room to see me still bent over holding the bar of weights. They eventually were able to pry the weights out of my hands, and then they slid me onto a board. I was screaming the whole time. It then took eight full grown men to lift me up from the floor on the board to the gurney. They were all such gentlemen. None of them even made me feel like I was a big person. They were so awesome! I rode to the hospital in the ambulance. While I waited in the emergency room the next five hours, they gave me morphine every 20 minutes to dull the pain.

The doctor who first saw me had a hard time understanding exactly how I got injured. I could have told him that I was lifting weights, and my back went out. No, this was not enough. I was slightly high from the morphine, and I had to give him the whole story.

So there I was in my hospital gown and my new white Nike tennis shoes telling the doctor all about the *Body for Life* program. I stressed to him that I did not want this injury to stop me from continuing my exercise program. The doctor must have been inspired about my story, because he told me to just stop lifting the weights for a while, but it was still okay to continue with my cardiovascular exercise of walking. He said to continue walking on the treadmill as long as it didn't hurt my back. Within two weeks my back was back to normal, and I was back to a full workout with the weights.

We followed the Bill Phillips' program faithfully for about a year. I was able to lose 140 pounds, and was now down to 311 pounds.

In 2000 we took our first Disney World vacation. It had been about six weeks since I lost more than a pound or two. I was staying pretty steady, and I wasn't gaining any weight. We both did our workouts on the first day we arrived in Florida, but by dinner that night we had determined we had earned this vacation, so we decided that we would just eat freely and not work out. We rationalized that we would be walking a lot every day, so this would be more than enough to compensate for not working out. Believe it or not, I was actually shocked when we returned home from our 10 day vacation and I had gained 18 pounds.

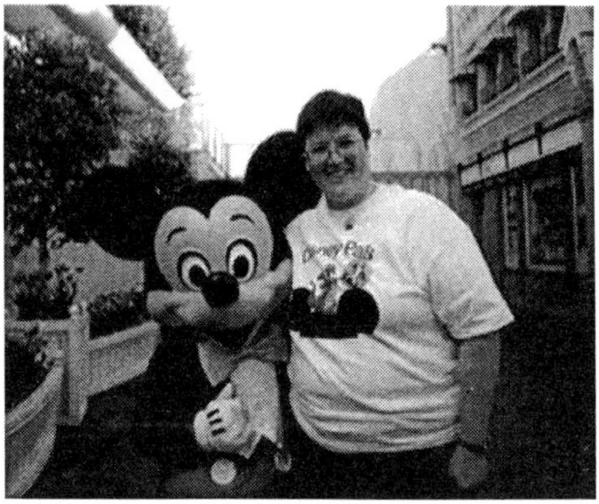

I was down 140 pounds from following Body for Life.
I weighed 311 pounds.

Over the next six months upon our return from our Disney World vacation, we found ourselves routinely skipping exercise days, until eventually we stopped exercising all together. Even though we stopped exercising, we still ate as outlined in *Body for Life*. We just did not exercise.

Dale and I still use the same principles from *Body for Life* for eating today. I will expand on this in a later chapter dealing with nutrition.

Because of my size, I ended up doing the 12 week challenge 3 times in row, and I was able to loose a total of 140 pounds. I know if I would have stuck with Bill Phillips' eating and exercise program long enough I would have lost all my weight, and would have been proud of the results. But I did not, and I began to gain weight.

Chapter 8

I Let Myself Go!

Over the next three years we did not include exercise as a part of our daily routine, and I gained about one to four pounds a month over this time. I did not weigh myself during this time, and pretty much felt I was staying about the same weight. The weight gain was very insidious.

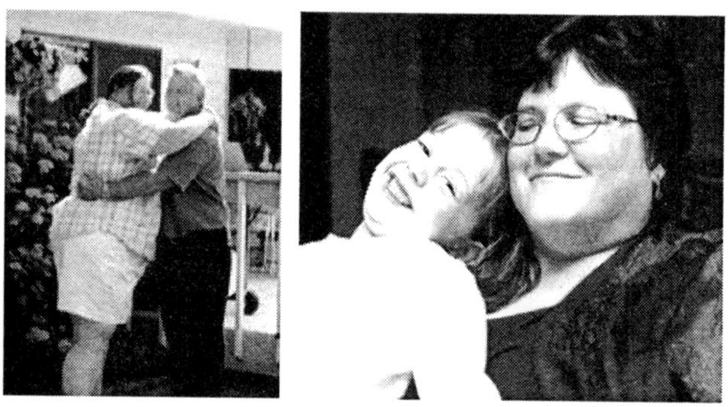

Dale and I in 2000 and my granddaughter Kelly in 2001.

In 2003 I weighed myself, and I was 390 pounds, and my dress size had pretty much gone from a 28 to a hefty 36/38. I know what you're saying, "How could you change that many dress sizes and not notice you were gaining weight.

I was using that same old Jedi mind trick that I used when I told myself I was happy and comfortable to be heavy. Every time I would change a dress size, I would just say to myself, *"Oh, that is weird; they must be making a different cut for this style."* I really had no idea that I was gaining a bunch of weight until I had jumped five dress sizes. I really felt I was maintaining my weight.

Dress sizes should not have been the only indicator that I was gaining weight. A year earlier in 2002, my really good friend Dana sat me down on our Disney Cruise vacation and said she was worried about me. She told me she loved me, and she wasn't ready to lose a really good friend. She told me I was really starting to look great in 2000, and she felt I was now going in the wrong direction. I admire her friendship, and the day she said those words to me. Not many people will speak that honestly to an obese friend. BRAVO to you, Dana! To this day, I keep those words close to my heart.

Dress sizes and worried statements from a friend were still not the only indicators that I was once again gaining weight. The pain I felt in my feet should have been like a brick hitting me in the head. I dealt with foot pain most of my obese life, but it always got severe as I went above the 400 pound mark.

You see, I stand all day at work, and there would be times when I would come home from work and just recline because my feet hurt so badly. That would pretty much be the end of my day. I would just sit back in a recliner and give my feet relief. Needless to say my social life came to a complete halt. If you wanted to visit with me, it would be by a phone call.

In the spring of 2002 my feet got really bad, and the pain became so extreme, I did not know if I was going to be able to continue to work. I went to a doctor, and I was told that the extreme pain was caused by bunions (otherwise known as hallux valgus) and a hammer toe (which is a deformed toe, shaped like a hammer). Hallux valgus is a sometimes painful structural deformity of the bones and the joint between the foot and big toe. Basically my second toe stuck up from the rest of my toes and rubbed up against my shoes and other toes.

The solution was to have surgery on both feet. In June of 2002 the doctor removed the knuckle on the second toe of the left foot and inserted a pin to hold it together. On my big toe they removed a bunion from the side and removed bone from that toe to restructure it. They added three screws during the reconstruction that remain today.

In October 2002 they did the same surgery to the other foot. They also had to correct the original surgery on my left foot because my toe was now sticking straight up. One of the tendons was not reattaching itself correctly.

Bless my Mom's heart, she came to Idaho from Seattle and stayed with me for both surgeries. She literally waited on me hand and foot. Thank You!

Okay, sorry for the graphic detail. For the most part the surgery took away the pain, and I was able to stay on my feet all day once my feet heeled. If you were to ask me, I would say the foot problem was caused by my excessive weight. However, the doctor did say this happens to skinny people too.

Looking back at the time period I was severely obese (above 300 pounds), it seems like there was always pain in my feet, knees, back, and hips. My mom said all of the above ran in our family. However, I knew the reason I hurt, and it was not hereditary.

I recall two stories that stuck in my head around this time period. The first involved my youngest stepdaughter, Lisa. All the kids and grandkids were sitting around a room at Christmas, and Lisa commented, *"It is very remarkable how well you get around for someone of your size, considering most people your size are bedridden."*

My sister Johnnie told me about an argument my niece had with a friend. It was about whose aunty's butt was bigger. She was very serious about winning this argument. She would stand up with her hands on her hips convinced that her aunt had the biggest butt.

As much as this was meant as a compliment from Lisa, both these comments really got me thinking about my size, and how others might see me. As most fat people know, you do not see yourself as fat or as big as other people may view you.

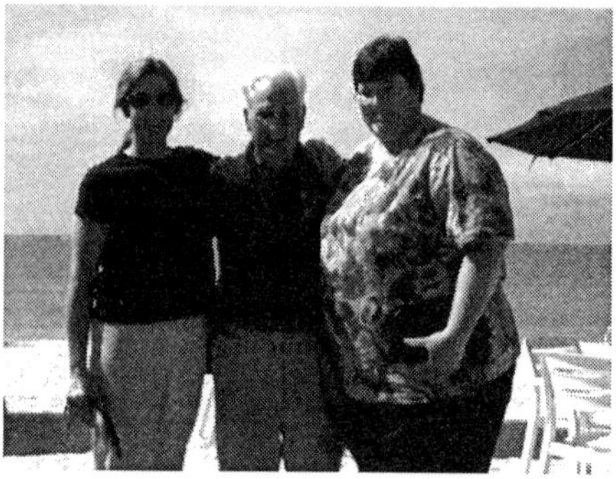

Top: my sister Johnnie and Uncle Brooks.
Bottom: Johnnie and Cousin Kitten,
2003 – Back to 390 pounds.

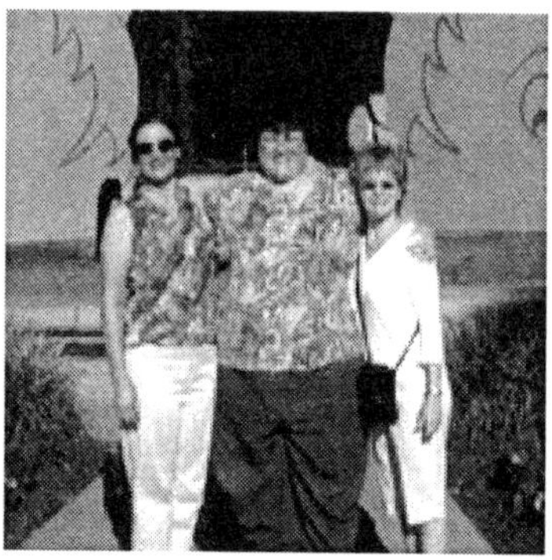

Chapter 9

My Last Chance

Early in 2002, I remember seeing a television commercial for Gastric Bypass Surgery. It featured Carnie Wilson, my fellow Weight Watchers campmate. I said to myself, *"Well, it looks like she fixed her weight problem."* I was happy for her; she looked great.

I recall researching Gastric Bypass but it was not covered under the insurance I had at the time, so I did not dig too deeply. At that time, I could not afford the surgery out of my pocket.

Toward the end of 2003, however, my company's insurance changed, and the new insurance did cover this procedure, so I began my research.

I weighed 390 pounds plus or minus as my research began. I had spent my whole life dieting, and doing one weight loss program after another, always failing to actually correct my weight problem. As a matter of fact, it seemed every time I did a diet, I just ended up weighing more than I did when I started it.

I looked at Gastric Bypass as MY LAST CHANCE! This was my last chance to get it right. In my mind, the amount of weight I needed to lose was just not feasible with a diet or traditional weight loss program.

As I researched and studied the procedure, I found that the surgery is only one part (or one tool in the shed) used to ultimately reach a permanent weight loss goal. It would take a multiple-prong commitment to eating properly, supplementing with vitamins, and exercising properly. A failure to commit to all, and a change for a lifetime, would ultimately be a failure of the Gastric Bypass Surgery.

The envelope of time for effective weight loss after Gastric Bypass Surgery is 12 to18 months. Which means whatever your weight loss, you need to try to lose it within that 12 to18 month period. After that time period, you can still lose weight, but your stomach does stretch over the 18 months, so it is harder to lose additional weight. After your stomach stretches, you do not have the sense of fullness like you did right after the surgery. Typically, most Gastric Bypass patients will lose 60-80 percent of their excess weight in this time period. I will talk a little more about the actual surgery later in the book and show you an illustration.

Even though my insurance covered the surgery, I still had to come up with $5,800 out of pocket. Depending on the surgeon your amount may very, but my financial responsibility was $1,800.00 down, and I made payments on the remaining $4,000.00.

I started my research on the following website, and highly recommend you start here too.

http://www.obesityhelp.com

I found this website offers the most support to find doctors, hospitals, and how to deal with your insurance. It is totally filled with testimonials from patients. These testimonials are not only about their surgery and weight loss experiences, but their testimonials are about different doctors and hospitals doing this procedure.

This was really helpful to me during my research. I was able choose a doctor, and read every patient's journey with that doctor. This made me feel very comfortable during the selection process.

I found that one of the most important factors in choosing a doctor, besides a long list of successful surgeries, is a doctor with a monthly or bi-monthly support group. It is best if you attend this support group pre and post-operation. I will discuss more about support groups later in the book.

In the spring of 2004 I made an appointment for my initial consultation. I spent two to three months reading every profile under this doctor. So I was pretty fixated about getting as much information as I could.

It took a month to get the appointment. I finally got in on June 3, 2004. By the time I walked in the door for this consultation, my mind was already made up. I was going to do the surgery unless this surgeon talked me out of it for some kind of health reason. It was kind of weird at first because I felt like I already knew this surgeon. By now, I had already read all the different profiles on his site 10 times over.

I was super impressed with my first visit. He spent two hours talking with me and he answered all my concerns and questions. Not only did he answer my questions, he also talked to me about the life-changing aspects of the surgery. He stressed in this initial meeting that Gastric Bypass was not a miracle cure, and I was going to have to do my part to make it work. He did say, "Gastric Bypass is just a tool to a healthier life, but without other life changes and commitments, the surgery could fail."

First and foremost, after surgery I would have to make the proper food choices for the rest of my life. The first year would be made up of a very restrictive diet, but as other foods were introduced, I would have to make the right food choices. I am lucky that I found the *Body for Life* program when I did, because it became my model of making the right food choices. It was very important to consume lean protein, good carbohydrates, and healthy fats.

With Gastric Bypass you must also supplement your food with vitamins because the absorption of critical vitamins is diminished after the bypass.

You must be able to commit to a lifetime of supplementing your diet. You will have to take a multiple vitamin with iron, calcium/magnesium, and possibly B-12 after the first year, and you will have to continue these supplementations for the rest of your life.

You must also be dedicated to a healthy fitness program for the rest of your life. This happens to be the most important tool in my life-changing commitments. As you know from my previous diets and weight loss programs, this was the first thing I stopped doing once the weight came off. This time around, I promised myself that I would not ever give up on the fitness. I was ready to make a total commitment.

My doctor stressed this three-prong approach (Surgery, Proper Food & Supplementation, and Fitness) during our initial consultation, and said that I would have to sign a contract that highlighted these three subjects before he would agree to do surgery on me. Basically, you would set yourself up for failure if you were not totally committed to all.

At the end of our initial meeting he also gave me a book called *Weight Loss Surgery: Finding the Thin Person Hiding inside You*, by Barbara Thompson. I ended up reading this book cover to cover more than once. It was very informative and provided many details about the operation. The book also explained the possible complications, as well as the successes of, Gastric Bypass Surgery. The book contained half a dozen or so testimonials. I definitely recommend, after reading my book, that you take a look at this book too.

At the end of our first meeting, I pretty much had already decided I was going to do it, so we went ahead and scheduled a surgery date for July 26th at 10:00 a.m. Of course, this was pending insurance approval. I was told it would take approximately three weeks to receive approval, and if the insurance did not approve it, then I would have to reschedule the surgery.

I spent the next three weeks on pins and needles waiting for that insurance approval. I went into major depression on several occasions worrying about the insurance not going through. It actually only took 15 days to approve the surgery, but I had to wait an extra week because I never received an approval letter. I called on the 16th, and they told me it was still pending. I called back on the 24th and they said I had been approved on the 17th. Because I never got the approval letter I spent an extra week worrying. My advice is to follow up daily after your first two weeks to help save the extra stress.

Yes!! Finally I was approved!

Because I did not want to gain more weight, if the surgery was not approved, I barely ate waiting for the news. That probably added to my depression.

Chapter 10

The Last Supper

Even though I had read as much as possible about Gastric Bypass Surgery, and I had an initial visit with my surgeon, I still was not sure about what I was going to be able to eat once I had the surgery done. There are very strict rules concerning what you can and cannot eat the first year. But eventually you can start eating most of the same foods you did prior to surgery, just without high levels of sugar. Everyone is different and some may be able to eat what others cannot. I was not aware of this at the time, or it did not click back then, that eventually one day you would be able to eat pretty much the same as prior to the surgery. I was under the impression that the strict first year rules would apply forever, so I began what I called my last supper.

With one month until the surgery, I felt a need to sample every food just one last time. This was because I had a fear of not being able to eat that food again after surgery. So I spent the next four weeks eating all my favorite meals for the last time. I still had to fight this overeating urge for the next four weeks, and I was quite surprised that I only gained 12 pounds. Because I ate a lot!

One of the most difficult tasks anyone will go through while waiting for the Gastric Bypass Surgery, is writing dear family and friends letters.

This was recommended in the weight loss surgery book I read and recommended in the last chapter. It suggested that you write a letter to family members and friends just in case something happened during your surgery. I wrote one letter to my family and one letter to my friends. Because there are no guarantees in life, and something could go wrong during the surgery, you should have a letter to family and friends ready to be sent.

It was explained to me that there was a risk of infection, allergic reactions, disfiguring scars, severe loss of blood, loss (or loss of function) of any organ, brain damage, cardiac arrest, or death. In addition to these risks, there was also the possibility of additional surgery required because of complications of the first surgery. So having this letter in case something happens is important.

I spent about two weeks thinking about what to say in these two letters. I prayed over and over for God's help in wording these letters just right. I will put these letters at the end of this chapter so you can get an idea how these letters may be written.

As my surgery drew close, I had one final pre-op meeting with my doctor six days before the scheduled surgery.

This meeting was heavily focused on my lifetime commitment to the surgery. In sports this would be called a final gut check. No pun intended. This was the final confirmation before I had the surgery.

The first subject in our meeting was the **Request and Informed Consent Form**. This form covered the following:

Request and Informed Consent

DO NOT SIGN THIS FORM UNTIL YOU HAVE READ IT FULLY AND UNDERSTAND ITS CONTENTS

Patients Name: Anita-Nell Swanson **Date:** 7/21/04

The following has been explained to me in general terms and I understand that:

- **My Diagnosis:** Clinically Severe Obesity
- **Nature Of Procedure:** Laparoscopic Roux-en-Y Gastric Bypass and possibly Open Roux-en-Y Gastric Bypass if necessary.
- **Purpose:** The purpose of this procedure is to reduce weight from Severe Obesity.
- **Material Risk of Procedure:** Includes risk of infection, allergic reactions, disfiguring scars, severe loss of blood, loss (or loss of function) of any organ, brain damage, cardiac arrest, or death.
- **In Addition to These Material Risks:** There may be other possible risks involved in this procedure, including but not limited to: conversion to an open procedure, leak from intestine requiring re-operation. Re-operation due to intestinal or metabolic complications.

- **Likelihood of Success of the Above Procedure:** (Good) (Fair) (Poor) Mine was checked off as Good

- **Practical Alternatives to This Procedure Include:** Open Procedure/Diet/Exercise

- **If I Choose Not to Have the Above Procedure, My Prognosis (Future Medical Conditions) is:** Continued Obesity.

I understand that the physician, medical personnel and other assistants will rely on statements about the patient, the patient's medical history, and other information in determining whether to perform the procedure or the course of treatment for the patient's condition and in recommending the procedure which has been explained.

I understand that the practice of medicine is not an exact science and that NO GUARANTEES OR ASSURANCES HAVE BEEN MADE TO ME concerning the results of this procedure. I also consent to diagnostic studies, tests, anesthesia, x-ray examinations, and any other treatment or courses of treatment relating to the diagnosis or procedure described herein.

I also consent to any tissues, specimens, or organs removed from the patient's body in the course of any procedure being tested or retained for scientific purpose and then disposed of within the discretion of the physician, facility or other health care provider.

I also understand I have been advised not to become pregnant after bariatric surgery until my weight has stabilized.

I also understand that if my procedure is performed videoscopically, the use of trocars, instruments and energy sources may result in injury to the organs such as: stomach, bowel, kidney, bladder, spleen, reproductive organs and/or major blood vessels, lungs, esophagus, common bile duct. This may require additional surgery to repair. I understand that my procedure may involve the use of permanent implantable medical devices (whose long term effects may be unknown) and may subsequently result in injury and require additional surgery or treatment.

BY SIGNING THIS FORM, I ACKNOWLEDGE

- THAT I HAVE READ OR HAD THIS FORM READ AND/OR EXPLAINED TO ME
- THAT I FULLY UNDERSTAND ITS CONTENTS
- THAT QUESTIONS HAVE BEEN ANSWERED SATISFACTORILY. ALL BLANKS OR STATEMENTS THAT I DO NOT APPROVE OF WERE STRICKEN BEFORE I SIGNED THIS FORM.

I also have received additional information including, but not limited to, the materials listed below related to the procedures described herein.

I hereby voluntarily request and consent to the performance of the procedures described or referred to herein by Dr. W. C. Oakley and any other physicians or medical personnel who may be involved in the course of my treatment.

______________________ ______________________

Witness Date Patient Signature Date

Wow! There is a mouthful. I got a sense of fear as I read this form. The word "**death**" stuck out larger than any word on the form. However, instead of second guessing my emotions, I fell back on my faith, and I remembered that God already knows my days are numbered, and the choice that I make today is how I am going to live out the rest of those days.

I can either live every day that God gives me on this earth feeling healthy from the inside out, or worry about how I am going to tie my shoes in the morning.

A side note: *(When my youngest daughter moved out, this was her biggest fear for me. She said, "How are you going to tie your shoes when I am gone, since I have been doing it for you over the past two years." My daughter moved out, when I was at my highest weight of 527 pounds.)*

So I felt with this procedure, I was moving forward to being healthier from the inside out. I then signed and dated this form and we moved on to the **Binding Obesity Contract**

I called this contract my **Commitment Contract.**

W.C. OAKLEY, M.D. F.A.C.S.
Diplomat, American Board of Surgery
General Surgery/Bariatric
333 N 1st Suite 120
Boise, Idaho 83703

BINDING OBESITY CONTRACT

With __Anita-Nell Swanson__ and W. Christian Oakley, M.D.

This contract is written solely for the benefit of the patient to assist them in obtaining the best results possible after "Obesity Surgery." Surgery alone does not work in reducing weight and requires lifelong and significant changes in habits. The patient agrees to abide by and adhere to the following principals:

1. To eat only to the point of feeling full or satisfied.

2. To avoid frozen, soft or melted ice cream, junk food and high calorie liquids.

3. To have NO calories between meals. A set mealtime is the only time for calories.

4. To see a Counselor or Psychiatrist if Dr. Oakley suggests it.

5. To keep follow-up appointments as recommended by Dr. Oakley.

6. To utilize Vitamin and Calcium supplements for

life, and be monitored with blood work and physical exams for life.

7. Exercise 5 days per week for 30 minutes beginning 3 weeks after surgery.

BY SIGNING THE CONTRACT I AM ACKNOWLEDGING THAT I FULLY UNDERSTAND THE ABOVE AND AGREE TO ADHERE TO ALL OF THE ABOVE.

PATIENT: ________________________ Date: __________

WITNESSED: _____________________ Date: __________

As I read through this contract, I said to myself, *"This seems pretty straightforward, and I know in my heart that I can do it."* I was very serious about this commitment, and making my permanent life change.

Now two and a half years later and looking back:

- Have I missed taking my vitamins more than 1 day? **Yes.**
- Has there been a week that I only exercised 3 or 4 days? **Yes.**
- But have there also been other weeks that I exercise 7 days in a row? **Yes.**
- Have I on very, very rare occasions eaten a TCBY frozen yogurt? **Yes.**

For the most part I have stuck to the contract as written, and I believe these are excellent rules to follow and will lead to a healthy life.

After signing the Commitment Contract, I was required to take an Obesity Surgery Patient True or False Exam.

I was told by Jennifer, who was administering the True or False exam, that if I did not pass this exam, they would have to cancel my surgery. After I took the exam, she said that she was just joking about the pass or fail; they just wanted to make sure each patient had a clear understanding of the surgery.

What follows is the exam, and the answers I gave are in bold.

W.C. OAKLEY, M.D. F.A.C.S.
Diplomat, American Board of Surgery
General Surgery/Bariatric
333 N 1st Suite 120
Boise, Idaho 83703

OBESITY SURGERY PATIENT EXAM

This examination is given to confirm you understand the information we discussed on surgical treatment options for severe obesity:

All questions are True/False. Circle your response.

1. **TRUE**/FALSE - Surgery for severe obesity is an option after failure of medical treatment (dieting, behavioral or exercise programs).
2. **TRUE**/FALSE - Obesity Surgery can be performed by an open incision or by laparoscopic technique.
3. **TRUE**/FALSE - Obesity Surgery is an aide to dieting, and patients may not lose weight.
4. **TRUE**/FALSE - Patients can die as a result of surgery for obesity.
5. **TRUE**/FALSE - Patients after obesity surgery need vitamin and mineral supplements and periodic nutritional assessments for life.
6. **TRUE**/FALSE - Some Patients require additional surgery for complications after obesity surgery.
7. **TRUE**/FALSE - Nutritional problems may occur after obesity surgery, which may require hospitalization or even reversal of the obesity procedure.
8. TRUE/**FALSE** - Serious complications cannot occur with obesity surgery.

9. **TRUE**/FALSE - Persistent vomiting or diarrhea can occur after obesity surgery.
10. **TRUE**/FALSE - Laparoscopic obesity surgery is new and the long-term results are unknown at this time.

Patient Signature ________________ Date __________

Witness Signature ________________ Date __________

All three of the forms presented in this chapter were signed by me, witnessed by Dr. Oakley's assistant, Jennifer, and were dated 7-21-04. As you can see by now, the surgery was NOT just another run of the mill weight-loss program, and it takes a real commitment to do it with success. Otherwise you are just setting yourself up for failure.

The rest of the meeting was spent going over my financial responsibility, and a pamphlet reviewing the nutrition and Gastric Bypass Surgery guidelines (which I will cover in detail in the next few chapters). I was then sent off to have more blood work for the surgery.

As promised, here are the letters to my family and friends. The objective was to write both letters, and give them in a sealed envelope to a trusted person with instructions to open only upon death from complication of the surgery. The person I trusted with these letters was my friend Dana.

To My Dear Family,

I am writing this in case anything goes wrong with my surgery. I wanted to let you know that if I'm in Heaven it's okay. I knew going into this that God was with me and if something happened it was His will. I also believe that Jesus is my Savior, and He will be greeting me at Heaven's gates. So be happy for me.

I really love and care for you all. I look back over my life and realize how blessed I have been. Mom and Dad, you have always tried to support me and guide me in the right direction. Dale, who would have thought we could mix two families and have it all turn out so well. One of the best things I have ever done was to marry you, and I treasure each day I am with you. To Leah, Lisa, and Kristen: I am so thankful that you all have grown into beautiful adults and seem to be making good choices. My son-in-laws Ron, Shawn, and John: Thanks for being good husbands and dads. And to my precious grandkids: Go out and follow your hearts' passion and live life to the fullest. To my siblings Johnnie, Ed, and Alvin: We have had our ups and downs, and I feel closer to you all now than I ever have, Love you! To my extended family: You have all been by my side throughout my life, thanks.

I wish I had the courage to write individual notes to you all, but I don't.

Please celebrate my life!

Love forever, Anita-Nell

To My Dear Friends,

I am writing this in case anything goes wrong with my surgery. I wanted to let you know that if I'm in Heaven it's okay. I knew going into this that God was with me and if something happened it was His will. I also believe that Jesus is my Savior, and He will be greeting me at Heaven's gates. So be happy for me.

I really love and care for all of you, I look back over the last five years of my life and realize what a blessing you all have been. I have done some reflecting over the past few months and realize all the changes I have been through, and I know I could not have done it without my Disney Pals.

You all have been there for me in many different ways. From emails to phone calls, cards or letters, or hugs just when I needed them. I thank you! I thank all of you for sharing your lives with me; it was the best ride I could have ever hoped for. I found a true group of friends who have stuck with me through thick and thin. I wish I had the courage to write individual notes to you all, but I don't.

Please celebrate my life!

Love forever, Anita-Nell

It just so happened that when I was looking for the right words for my letters, and making plans for the surgery, I received the following letter from my daughter, Leah:

GIVING ME LIFE

Life is such a precious thing
And you so willing gave it to me.
On September 18th at 9:18

Down in California
High above the bay,
Well, hun, it's just you and me, kid,
That's what you would say.

Far from our family
Needing each other so much,
I was a small, little baby,
So soft to the touch

Together we have made it through
In times so near the end.
You're not only my Mother,
But my dearest friend.

Now is the time you need me most.
But I am so far away,
Before they put you under
Just close your eyes to see
Me standing there beside you,
Telling you everything is gonna be okay.

Then when you wake up
To a brand new life,
To celebrate good things
And see me as a wife

Sometimes I look back at my life
And choose to cry,
But the tears come from happiness
And all the love inside

So if our King, the Lord
Decides he wants you with Him instead,
You will always be the most wonderful,
The best Mother in my head.

But God knows I need you now
So here on earth you'll stay,
And being so afraid right now
I'll cherish you more each day.

I love you, Mom!

Leah

Chapter 11

Gastric Bypass Surgery

The term morbid obesity refers to patients who are 100 percent above -- or 100 pounds above -- their ideal body weight. In simple terms, it is defined as:

- BMI >=40 or
- Weighing at least twice the ideal weight, or at least 100 pounds more than ideal weight.

Morbid obesity greatly increases the chances of developing health conditions that can result in significant physical, mental and social disabilities. It can also cause death. Morbidly obese, as well as severely obese individuals, with a BMI of 40 or more with obesity-related health problems may be considered candidates for obesity surgery. *(Source: Obesityhelp.com)*

At my highest weight of 527 pounds, my BMI then was 71.4. On the day of my surgery I weighed 392 pounds and my BMI was 53.2.

(Figure 1) is an illustration of the Gastric Bypass, and the actual size that my stomach will be after the surgery.

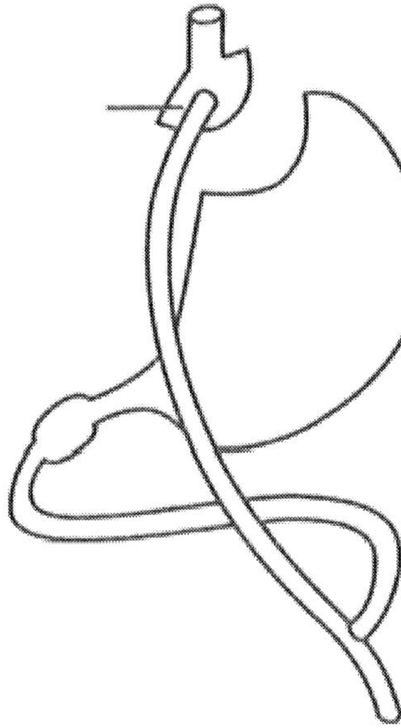

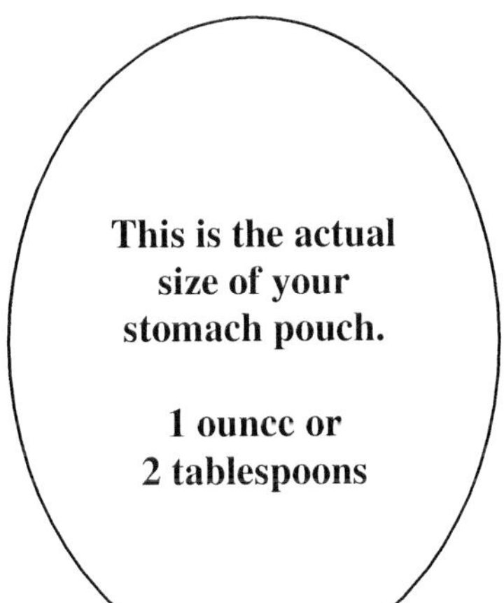

Figure 1

Weight loss after Gastric Bypass occurs primarily because of the limited amount of food one can eat. Calories are still absorbed after surgery so a healthy, low calorie diet must be followed. Appetite decreases significantly after surgery, which aids in controlling food intake.

Expected Weight Loss

*Most of the weight loss will be in the first 12-18 months after surgery. Patients typically lose about 40-50 percent of their current weight or 60-80 percent of excess body weight (*Figure 2*). Weight loss varies significantly from one patient to the next. NOT ALL PATIENTS LOSE 100 percent of excess weight and this is not possible without a healthy diet and consistent exercise routine.*

EXAMPLE:

Female 5ft. tall weighs	*300#*
Ideal weight	*100#*
Excess weight	*200#*
80% of excess weight	*160#*
Expected weight loss	*160#*

Figure *2*

SUCCESS:

For maintenance of long-term weight loss and weight loss of greater than 80 percent of excess body weight, patients must exercise, eat well, and supplement.

Ultimate success depends on the dedication of the three- prong approach in (Figure 3).

(Source of text, illustrations, and Figures 1, 2 & 3, from Dr. Oakley's hand out called "Nutritional Guidelines After Your Gastric Bypass").

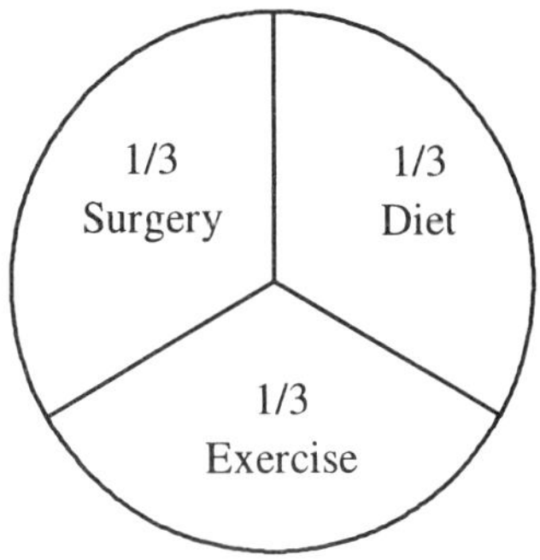

Figure 3

It is Monday, July 26, 2004. Today is my day! Up until now, I have lived with obesity for a majority of my life. I've tried diets, I've tried weight loss programs, I have been in pain, and I lost organs, all from being fat. Enough! I viewed this surgery as my last chance to get it right, and for me to become healthy from the inside out. I knew in my heart that Gastric Bypass Surgery was the only aid or way I was going to lose the amount of weight I needed to lose. I basically have 18 months from today to get it right, but more important; I am done with my past. I am going to make radical changes in my life, and this time, I am going to keep with the commitments, and make those changes permanent. This time, I am making these changes as a lifetime commitment, not just a weight loss commitment!

My metaphor for this surgery was the story I read when I was little about the queen who circled the earth with the ice cream planet in tow. I have often thought about this story throughout my life, and wished I was that thin and beautiful queen. Now is my opportunity to be that queen.

After taking 1-½ ounces of phosphor-soda yesterday to clean out my system, and drinking nothing but water, coffee, juice, or soup until midnight, I was finally on my way to the hospital. I was little nervous, but put it all in God's hands.

Dale and my Mom drove me to the hospital. I had to be there at 8:00 a.m. When I arrived, the nurses took me back and prepped me for surgery within half an hour of my arrival. I went into surgery right around 10:00 a.m. The surgery was done by Laparoscopy. They inserted their instruments and camera through 5 half inch holes in my abdomen. I recovered from this surgery quicker than any other surgery in the past.

I was out of surgery by 1:00 p.m. and in my room by 2:00 p.m. I was loaded from the anesthesia and pain killers until sometime late into the night. After that, I only remember being uncomfortable with pain.

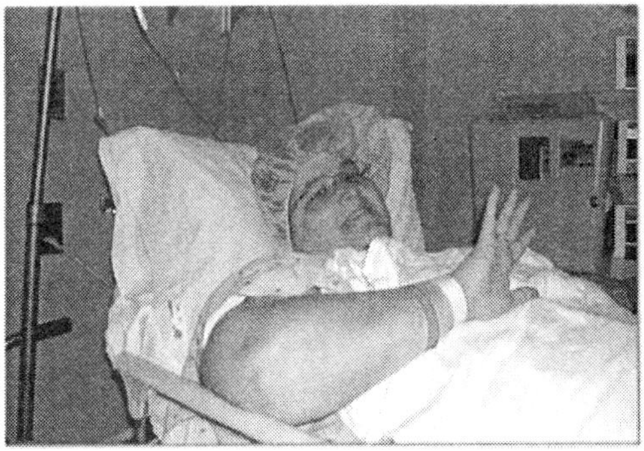

7-26-2004, 9:30 a.m., on my way to surgery.

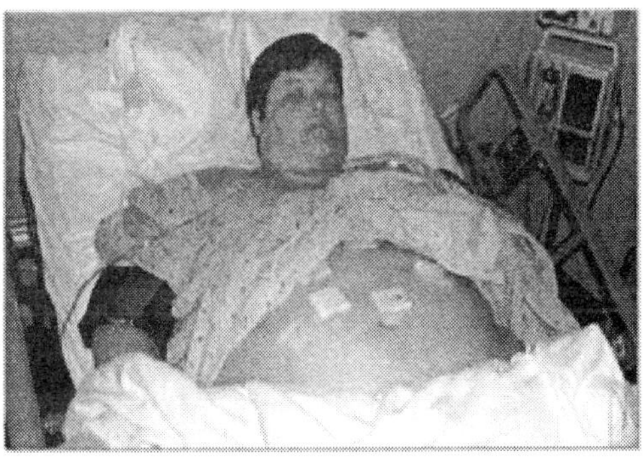

7-26-2004, 2:00 p.m., after my surgery.

My mom and Dale were the best supporters. They both stayed at the hospital the whole day of the surgery. My mom returned the following two days to be with me, and Dale came to visit right after work.

The first thing Tuesday morning, I got up and took a shower. It was painful at first to get moving, but it felt so good to get cleaned up. I visited with my surgeon after my shower, and he assured me that the surgery was perfect, and could not have gone any better. He also said that the next day, Wednesday, I would be taking a leak test. If all went okay from the test, and none of my organs leaked, then I could start eating. Really, this was the furthest thing from my mind at the time. His departing words to me were that my wounds were healing nicely, and the rest was up to me.

And it was up to me, I thought to myself. I was the only one who could make or break this surgery, and I was confident that I had made the correct first step, and now the rest of the life-changing commitments would follow.

After my surgeon left the room, I was up and out of bed, and down the hall for my first walk. I was a little stiff and in mild pain, but it was time to get the body moving and circulating. My first walk lasted about 20 minutes. The nurses calculated that 19 laps around the 6th floor was one mile. By the end of the second day, I had walked two more times. I had put in the 19 laps for one mile. Not bad, I thought! I spent the rest of the day calling family and friends and napping between walks.

On the third day I had the leak test, and passed with flying colors. When I came back from my first walk of the day, I got my first post-surgery meal. It consisted of a red or cherry flavored Popsicle™, green Jell-O™, and a small bowl of broth. That was one of the best Popsicles™ I ever had. I had a few spoonfuls of broth, and then I was full.

This was the first time in my life I remembered feeling full. It was kind of weird since I never really felt this before. After lunch I went for another walk. At the end of my second walk, I had already hit the one mile mark.

I met with the dietitian, Jennifer, later that day. She talked to me about all the supplements I needed to take in my new life. I asked her about salt, and she said not to worry about it because I would not be able to eat enough to exceed the salt intake. She told me I was not going to eat much, so I had to be sure to consume 60 grams of protein, a multivitamin, and lots of water every day.

I walked again later that afternoon. After the walk, my doctor came and said, "Do you want to stay another night?" I told him I felt fine, and I would go home. So I was discharged.

So for the surgery, everything went well. I know not everybody has, or will have the same results, but my doctor did say my surgery was pretty typical of the average Gastric Bypass Surgery.

I was discharged with the following instructions from my doctor:

POSTOPERATIVE INSTRUCTIONS AFTER OBESITY SURGERY

These instructions will serve as general guidelines to assist you in your recovery after surgery for severe obesity. If you have a question or problem, do not hesitate to call our office for instructions.

Discharge Instructions:

1. Check temperature twice daily for the first week – call if fever is 101 or higher.
2. You may bathe or shower; do not scrub incisions for 3 weeks.
3. Notify us if redness or drainage from incisions occurs.
4. Contact us for vomiting or diarrhea, which lasts more than 24 hours. If possible, call during office hours so we can address the issues.
5. Use the incentive spirometry bottle four times daily for 10 days.
6. Walk daily until you can walk 30 minutes at a time. Several walks each day is better.
7. Increased gas is common the first 3-6 weeks; we recommend Gas-x or Digel for relief.
8. Do not take any anti-inflammatory pain medications unless approved by Dr. Oakley, i.e. ibuprofen, Advil, Motrin, Naprosyn, Aleve.
9. Take vitamin-calcium supplement daily; Flintstone™ Chewables with iron. Three Tums™ daily for calcium

POST-OP DIET INSTRUCTIONS

The post-op diet is divided into three stages to allow a gradual adjustment.

Stage I Liquid diet for 2 weeks with 2-3 protein drinks per day.

STAGE I FIRST 2 WEEKS POST – OP

Liquids only from list below 3 times daily at set times. Liquid protein drinks 2-3 times a day for your meals.

Remember: small amounts (4-6 ounces)

Go slowly (30 minutes to drink 6 ounces).
When you feel full STOP.
No carbonated drinks for 4 weeks.

LIQUID DIET

- Fruit juice
- Crystal Light, NutraSweet Kool-Aid
- Diet drinks
- Broth
- Blenderized soup
- Skim or Lactaid milk
- Sugar-free Jell-O™ or Popsicles™
- Yogurt
- Sugar-free pudding
- Cottage cheese

– Applesauce, oatmeal, Cream of Wheat

PROTEIN SUPPLEMENTS: Designer protein from GNC, Carnation Instant Breakfast, Ensure, Boost, Sustacal, or any protein powder supplement from a health food store.
These are best mixed with skim milk or Lactaid milks as lactose intolerance can occur the first few weeks after surgery. The protein powder can also be mixed with yogurt or with fruit and fruit juice if blenderized. **Remember: Protein is needed for healing, maintenance of muscle, and energy.**

I really only got to eat one meal in the hospital, so I did not have much practice when I arrived home. It was a whole new way of eating, especially at first. I kind of winged it.

I had done a little grocery shopping prior to the surgery. I had bought some sugar-free Jell-O™, sugar-free Popsicles™, carb control yogurt, protein shakes, and several kinds of soup which you could throw into a blender. They call that blenderized soup. I also bought some baby spoons. These are nice because when you only eat an ounce or two of soup, you can stretch it out using these spoons.

Food would go much further now. A can of soup could be served over a couple of days to a week. As I opened a new can of soup, I would blenderize what I needed for my meal, and put the rest in the refrigerator. I also did this with my protein shakes,

Jell-O™, and yogurt. I only discarded the Popsicles™ if I couldn't finish them.

In between the meals and snacks, I was able to drink water. The golden rule was you could not drink water 15 minutes before you ate a meal or snack, and half an hour after you ate.

Basically you spent the day eating and drinking during first three weeks.

I never got hungry for the first year. Not even hunger pains. I had to schedule to eat, and then I followed the schedule. Otherwise I might not get enough protein, or I would get dehydrated, and then I would feel sick.

So everything went fine for the first day at home. However, on Friday we had to take my mother-in-law, Maryann, to the emergency room, and found out she'd had a heart attack.

This was my first major crisis after my surgery. She was my mom away from my own mother. She had lived with Dale and me for the past 4 years. I wasn't prepared for eating during a crisis, and hadn't been warned about the necessity of taking care of myself.

The doctors ran tests on Maryann over the weekend, and decided she had to have quadruple bypass surgery. She remained in the hospital, in and out of consciousness after the surgery for the next four weeks, and eventually passed away within a month. I found out after this first weekend crisis, that I was ill prepared as it related to my nutritional health and hydration. I forgot that I was supposed to eat and drink regularly during the day. All my thoughts were with Maryann, and not on taking care of myself. I became very ill and nauseous because I did not eat or hydrate as I should. I ended up becoming very weak and sick by the end of the weekend. Dale said, "We need to take care of you, so you do not end up back in the hospital too."

By Monday I began planning my day by packing my daily meals on the go which included my hydration and supplements. I learned from this experience that you never know where life is going take you, and you should always be prepared. To this day, I pack my daily meals, just in case I get distracted from my daily routine. That way; I still have a meal ready.

My advice to all weight loss individuals, especially Gastric Bypass Surgery patients, is always be prepared with your daily meals and supplements, and do not rely on others for your nutritional needs.

For example, when you are on the run, you may find yourself at a restaurant which has nothing you can eat on the menu. You need to have a back-up plan. This is why you need to take accountability for your new life. Always be prepared, and have a meal ready to eat.

In the past when faced with a crisis, I would emotionally eat my way though that crisis. Now I did not have this option. I had to focus on the crisis without eating. I knew then that I would have to work through my emotions without eating for my comfort. It was whole new experience, and to this day, it is a thought in the back of my head when things get rough. You just have to refocus your thoughts elsewhere, and not fall back on eating.

Chapter 12

Eating and Nutrition

A majority of the information in this chapter is from Dr. Oakley's informational guidelines. I have responded to this information with my own personal experiences, and I have highlighted those experiences and/or comments in *italics* throughout this chapter.

Eating Methods After Gastric Bypass

What to Expect after Surgery:

After a Gastric Bypass you will need to make changes to your eating patterns. After surgery the diet progresses from a liquid diet to a soft diet and then to a modified regular diet. The diet progression is designed to allow you to heal. Initially, it helps you meet your protein and liquid needs and later, to meet your nutritional needs. It is important that you follow the diet progression to maximize healing and minimize risk for complications. The size of your stomach after surgery is about 1 ounce or 2 tablespoons. By six months after surgery, it may stretch to 8 ounces or 1 cup. Over the long term, the size of your stomach is likely to be 8-12 ounces or 1 to 1-1/2 cups. This will limit the amount of food you can eat at one time.

To successfully maintain a healthy weight and prevent weight gain, you must develop and keep healthy eating habits. You will need to be aware of the volume of food you can tolerate at one time and make healthy food choices to ensure maximum nutrition with minimum volume. Exercise must be a part of your daily routine as well.

After a few months I realized that you can't make up your nutritional nccds by grazing all day for a skipped meal. What I mean is that **you cannot try and make up for a lost meal by eating small amounts during the day in between your snack and meals**. You need to plan your meals.

Long-Term Eating Goals:

Swallowing food in chunks may block the stoma and prevent foods from passing into the intestine.

It is critical that you eat slowly and chew food well to lower the risk for getting anything caught in this area. The following tips may help you eat more slowly.

- ✓ Set aside 20-30 minutes to eat each meal.
- ✓ Take small bites of food. Using a smaller spoon and a saucer instead of a plate can help with portion control.
- ✓ Pay attention to taste, learn to savor your food.
- ✓ Stop eating as soon as you are full (overeating even one ounce can cause you to vomit and can lead to stretching your pouch.

Having the proper time to eat is very important. I found with myself that during the day at work, I was not able to break at times for a full 30 minutes to eat. I have always struggled with making time to eat properly at work, and I recommend that no matter the time or schedule, you need to make your eating time a priority.

Feeling of Fullness

Learn to recognize when you are full. Indications of fullness may be:

- A pressure or fullness in the center of your abdomen or just below your rib cage.
- Feelings of nausea, regurgitation or heartburn.

As I said, when I was in the hospital was the first time in my life that I actually felt a sense of fullness. I found as I got this sense of fullness I would also start to sneeze. So this became my second indicator to stop eating. It always seems to be just two sneezes. I do not always eat to the point of fullness where I sneeze, but if I do, I definitely know when it is time to stop eating.

Vomiting

Vomiting may occur after Gastric Bypass Surgery. It is most often the result of eating inappropriately and rarely a complication of surgery.

Common Eating-Related Causes of Vomiting:

- Eating too fast.
- Not chewing food properly.
- Eating too much at one time.
- Eating solids foods too soon after surgery.
- Drinking liquids either with meals or right after meals.
- Eating foods that do not agree with you.

If vomiting occurs, review the above common reasons for vomiting; stop eating solid foods and sip clear liquids (diluted juice, broth, tea). If changing your eating pattern does not help and vomiting is frequent or persistent, contact the surgeon.

I found that I only vomited when trying something new or unfamiliar. An example of this was mainly when I went out to eat. I found that the sauces and marinades on meats tend to make me vomit. So I got in the habit of asking for meats cooked plain and with no sauce when I would go out. I hope this is a good tip for you. The only other times I had a problem was when I tried to introduce new foods too soon.

Meal Pattern/Balanced Diet

Patients must choose foods with good nutritional value. The quantity of food you are able to eat at a meal will be reduced, and therefore the quality should be increased. You will progress to eating three meals a day once you have recovered from surgery. Each meal should have protein source (such as eggs, cottage cheese, fish, poultry, beans, meat, and tofu). Limit fat intake. You must learn to read labels, and choose lower fat and lean protein foods. Avoid snacking. Snacking will add significant calories and keep you from losing weight. Avoid filling up on foods with little nutritional value. Eating foods from each of the five food groups will provide balance. You must get a maximum amount of nutrition in a minimum amount of food.

I have already cautioned you about grazing. Make sure your snacks are not empty calories. If you are exercising more than 30 minutes a day, you may want to contact your doctor. You may need a higher protein or carbohydrate food after exercise, depending on your individual workout. Let your doctor know what kind of workout you are doing, i.e., cardiovascular or weight training, and he will help recommend what is right for you.

Liquids/Hydration

Drink liquids between meals. Recommended beverages are skim milk, water, low or no calorie drinks.

Just a reminder, the golden rule is to hydrate 15 minute before a meal or snack and 30 minutes after.

Certain Foods May Be Difficult to Tolerate

Tolerance to food varies from one individual to the next. Common foods that patients cannot tolerate include red meat (particularly roasted meat), fresh bread, skin of fruits and vegetables, seeds and fibrous vegetables, such as celery, corn and sweet potato, membranes of oranges or grapefruit, fried foods, and in some cases milk.

With the exception of milk, all of the above gave me a bad feeling in my stomach when I first tried them, so I tended to avoid them. After one year, I re-introduced them one at a time until I could tolerate them without discomfort. As of today, I can tolerate all of them in my diet without any discomfort.

Do not avoid a food just because you vomit once after eating it. You may wish to wait a few weeks before trying it again. Tolerance to foods may improve with time.

Sometimes it may not be the food, but just the way you body is reacting on that day. So don't continue to avoid foods just because you have one bad reaction. Quick example: The first time I introduced chili into my diet (5-6 month mark), I had no negative reaction. It tasted so good! A few weeks later I had the chili again, and I vomited. I was so bummed out. But instead of avoiding it as a food that I could not have, I tried it again a couple of weeks later and it was fine. I have had it many times since without any negative reaction. So just because you have a negative reaction once, it may not be the food, but your body's reaction to other factors. Other factors may include chewing your food too fast, taking too large of bites, or too much of volume at one time.

Possible Nutrition Related Complications after Gastric Bypass:

Vitamin and Mineral Deficiencies

The absorption of certain vitamins and minerals changes because of the area of intestine that is being bypassed. All patients must take supplements daily for the rest of their lives in order to avoid deficiencies.

A chewable multivitamin is recommended the first eight weeks after surgery. After this, a multivitamin with iron is required daily. Patients need to take calcium, and possibly B_{12}, as well.

Possible deficiencies include:

Vitamin B12

Vitamin B_{12} is necessary for proper nerve impulse transmission. A low B_{12} level can result in low iron status or anemia and in permanent neurological damage. Most patients have B_{12} stores that will last up to 18 months after surgery but B_{12} supplements are recommended at about 12 months after surgery. B_{12} levels must be tested annually.

Iron

Iron is needed to keep blood strong and to prevent anemia. Supplemental iron is recommended once you are home from the hospital. A multivitamin with added iron should provide enough iron. Iron levels must be tested annually.

Calcium

Calcium is needed to build strong bones and prevent osteoporosis.

For the first year I took a multivitamin with minerals and a separate calcium chewable tablet. After my one-year check-up, the doctor determined that I needed to add B_{12} *to my diet. At my two-year check-up, my blood work showed I no longer needed the* B_{12} *because I was making such good food choices. I was on the high end of all vitamins.*

Hair Loss

Most patients will have some degree of hair loss in the first year after surgery. Rapid weight loss causes some state of malnutrition. One of the body's responses to malnutrition is hair loss. Eating enough protein and consistently taking the recommended doses of vitamin and mineral supplements will minimize hair loss. By one year after surgery, hair should be back to baseline.

Specific doses for supplements may vary from one patient to the next. Supplemental calcium, B_{12} **and a multivitamin with iron are recommended. Doses will be recommended in clinic.**

I did follow all the rules regarding supplementations; however, I started losing my hair on daily basis from 6 to 10 months. I returned to my baseline around 18 months. My entire life I had straight hair. It did take a little longer for my hair to grow back, but the bonus was it grew back naturally curly.

Dumping Syndrome

Dumping Syndrome is a reaction that can occur after eating foods or liquids high in sugar. If a concentrated dose of sugar is released into the intestine, it can cause lightheadedness, shaking, cramps, nausea, perspiration and weakness. These symptoms are most often followed by the rapid onset of diarrhea. Eating too fast or too much can also cause "dumping." It is extremely unpleasant and unpredictable, thus, patients must avoid concentrated sugar and fat in foods.

I have always avoided high amounts of sugar because I did not want to experience dumping. I was never told about this, but I found out that sugar alcohol does the same thing to me if I eat more than 4 grams at a time. It also gives me really bad gas. I found that when I want to treat myself to a non-sugar treat, I have to check the label to make sure there is no more than 4 grams of sugar alcohol. Otherwise I will experience dumping.

POST-OP DIET INSTRUCTIONS

The post-op diet is divided into three stages to allow a gradual adjustment.

- **Stage I -** Liquid diet for 2 weeks with 2-3 protein drinks per day.

- **Stage II** - Soft diet of 3 meals a day for 4 weeks with 2 protein supplements per day

- **Stage III** - Regular diet of 3 meals a day

Stage I is printed out in full back in Chapter 11

STAGE II – SOFT DIET FOR 3-6 WEEKS

Soft foods from the list below can now gradually be added to your diet:

1. Three meals a day with a liquid protein drink twice daily for two of the meals.
2. No liquids with meals if soft food is included. You must wait 30-40 minutes for the pouch to empty before drinking.
3. CHEW WELL. The food must be almost liquefied before swallowing.

SOFT DIET

– Soft fruit (banana, melon, strawberries)
– Cooked vegetables and fish
– Soft pasta (well chewed)
– Eggs
– Toast or crackers

Every individual will vary in each stage. For me in Stage II, pasta was too filling, and I was unable to eat any protein when eating pasta. So I did not eat pasta again until after the first year. Now I only eat it for the carbohydrate factor before a long run. Toast also made me too full, so I also avoided it for the first year. For the past year and half I have been eating half a sandwich every day for lunch with a yogurt or fruit.

<u>STAGE III – REGULAR DIET OF 3 MEALS A DAY AFTER 6 WEEKS</u>

Gradually add regular foods and remember:

NO SNACKS: eat only at meal times
NO LIQUIDS with meals
Avoid cheap calories*:

- Fats
- High calorie liquids
- Sweets, ice cream, junk food, cookies

Discontinue protein supplements.

SUMMARY

- Follow three-stage diet plan to allow gradual adjustment.
- Eat only at set meal time.
- Go slowly.
- Chew well.
- When you feel full: **STOP!**

*Liquids, junk food, and sweets do not relieve hunger! Only solid food which fills the pouch and empties slowly will relieve hunger.

Six Weeks Post-Operation & Beyond:

Food

- Be patient, progress slowly.
- Continue a soft diet. Progress to a regular diet over 6-12 weeks after surgery.
- Always chew well.
- Introduce new foods slowly. Use caution with raw fruits and vegetables and avoid the skin at first.
- Follow a low-fat and low-sugar diet.
- Include foods from all food groups. Check the Food Guide at the end to ensure you are meeting your needs.
- Remember that your tolerance to foods will be different that it was before surgery.

Meal Pattern

- Your long-term goal is 3 meals per day with limited or very light snacks. Long-term maintenance of weight loss requires a consistent meal pattern.
- Meals are about 4 ounces in volume by 8-10 weeks after surgery (this should take 30 minutes to eat), up to 8 ounces (1 cup) by 7-8 months and never larger than 1 ½ cup in volume long term.
- Take your time eating. Set aside at least 30 minutes for meals.
- Avoid snacking. Snacking leads to weight gain.

Liquids

- No liquids 15 minutes before meals and 30 minutes after meals.
- You may need some protein-based liquids in between meals to meet your protein goal.
- Avoid sweetened drinks and sodas.

Protein

- Maintain protein intake as your goal.
- Eat protein foods in each meal.
- Eating enough protein will decrease feeling hunger, which helps with weight loss.
- Keeping your protein intake at goal is important for the rest of your life to maintain health.

Tips for Success

Changing lifelong habits takes time. Selecting healthy foods, exercising and paying attention to eating habits will help ensure weight loss and maintenance.

In the first year after your operation, the size of your stomach pouch will limit your intake. You will eventually be able to tolerate larger volumes of foods. You must not eat the amount you tolerate but instead, learn to eat appropriate portions. What you tolerate should not dictate what you eat. Patients must develop good eating habits, must learn to choose foods wisely and must control their intake. If this is not achieved, weight loss will only be short term.

- **Portion control is critical.**
- **Regular meal times are essential.**
- **Limited snacking is recommended.**

Be sure to always take your time eating. Set aside 30 minutes for your meals and set regular meal times. Eat at the table, not in front of the television or on the run. Take food from home for work meals as often as possible.

Keep portions small. Eat your protein foods first as these will help you feel full sooner. Use a side plate for your meals. Use a baby spoon when you are eating and chew each bite at least 20 times. Stop eating when you feel pain or discomfort.

One tip I found helpful is to eat two bites of protein for every one bite of carbohydrate. That is how you get your protein in before you feel full.

The Future

After your Gastric Bypass, calories are still absorbed. The surgery simply restricts your stomach capacity for a short time; you must develop new eating habits. As mentioned previously, you will need to follow a low-calorie, low-fat, low-sugar diet for the rest of your life in order to keep weight off.

After this surgery, the average person needs 1200 calories or less per day. Male patients and patients who participate in daily activity may be able to eat more than this and maintain weight loss. Regardless, ALL patients must be aware of their caloric intake and their diet choices.

Behavior change is necessary. Changing old habits takes time and simply having surgery will not result in behavior change. You must be an active participant in behavior change.

All patients will lose weight in the first 6-8 months after surgery. Many will not continue to lose weight after this period of time and some will even gain this weight back. This can be referred to as the "honeymoon" stage. When this stage ends, weight loss slows and diet and exercise become critical for continued weight loss.

Attend support group meetings and keep in touch with other Gastric Bypass patients to stay motivated and on track with your diet and exercise routines. Research shows that those patients who attend support groups lose more weight and are more likely to keep it off.

Seek professional help for depression and behavior modification if needed.

Come to your follow-up appointments. See a dietitian regularly for continued support and encouragement of diet changes.

Take the surgery seriously; it is not a cosmetic one. We do not measure success on what your weight loss results are one year post-operation. True success is maintaining the weight loss. Our goal is for you to avoid regain of weight in 2, 5 or 10 years, to stay healthy, to avoid medical problems associated with obesity, and to maintain a healthy weight.

As I entered into Stage III, and got a good regular schedule of eating, I found myself in a familiar pattern. I started to equate this eating lifestyle to the Body for Life program. It had the basic guidelines that a Gastric Bypass patient needs. I ate three meals and two snacks a day. When I reached goal I added a third snack in order to stop losing weight.

I highly recommend the Body for Life book. It is very informational for both eating and exercise. And according to both Bill Phillips and Dr. Oakley, you are not on a diet; you are just eating as a normal person should.

Protein Foods

Make protein a priority in your diet. Read labels for grams of protein. By about three months after surgery, most people need between 50 and 65 grams of protein a day. Some may need more, depending upon weight and height.

(Be sure to follow your diet progression for liquids, puree and soft food protein foods.)

FOOD	1 SERVING IS:	AMOUNT OF PROTEIN PER SERVING
Milk Nonfat or 1%, soy or low lactose milk **Yogurt** Light (low sugar and fat)	1 cup (8 oz)	8-10 grams per cup Read food labels as protein content may vary.
MEAT and PROTEIN ALTERNATIVES	1 oz chicken, turkey, fish, beef, pork 1 oz low fat cheese ¼ cup cottage cheese 1 egg ¼ cup egg substitute ½ cup cooked dried beans (navy, pinto, black, kidney, etc.) ½ cup cooked dried chickpeas, black-eyed peas, lentils ½ cup or 4 oz tofu ¾ cup split pea, lentil or bean soup 1 cup low fat chowder	7 grams per serving **Read food labels.**

For example: 3 oz of cooked meat, fish or chicken is about the size of a deck of cards or the size of the palm of your hand.

Low Fat Eating

**Keep your fat intake to a minimum.
Fat is found naturally in foods,
so limit added fat.**

Reading Food Labels

- ✓ Always check the serving size at the top of the label.
- ✓ Read the number of grams of fat per serving and keep it to less than 5 grams per serving.
- ✓ Read the number of calories per serving.
- ✓ Compare food labels for those with lowest fat and lowest calories.

Be aware that some foods labeled as "Low Fat" products may be higher in calories. Often products that have less fat will have more sugar and more calories.

Preparing Foods

- ✓ Avoid frying.
- ✓ Grill, bake, broil, roast, steam, boil, and microwave.
- ✓ Take skin off chicken.
- ✓ Cut off all visible fat from meat.
- ✓ Use cooking sprays and non-stick pans.
- ✓ Use egg whites instead of whole eggs.

Eating Away From Home

- ✓ Use a side dish for your main course.
- ✓ Ask how the foods are prepared.
- ✓ Ask for sauces on the side so you can control your portions.
- ✓ Avoid fast food.

Shopping for Foods

- Buy lean cuts of meat.
- Choose low or nonfat dairy products.
- Try lower fat versions of foods. (Be sure to check the labels to see if the product is lower in fat and calories than the regular version.)

Serving Food

- Avoid high fat dressings, sauces, gravy, sour cream.
- Season food with spices; butter substitute or low/non fat dressings.

Daily Food Guide For Gastric Bypass Patients

This food guide is for those patients who are at least 3 months post-operation. You must always eat slowly and chew your food well.

Protein: **50-65 grams per day**	**Each of the following serving sizes has approximately 7 grams of protein:** • 1 oz chicken, turkey, beef*, fish, pork • 1 egg, ¼ cup egg substitute • 1 oz cheese • ½ cup dried beans, peas or lentils • tofu (check label) • ¼ cup cottage cheese • 2 tbsp. peanut butter *(*Red meat may be difficult to tolerate.)*
Milk and Yogurt **2-3 servings per day**	**1 serving is:** • 8 oz of non-fat, 1% milk or soy milk • 8 oz of "light" yogurt (low in fat and sugar) *(Milk and yogurt also provide protein)*

<table>
<tr><td>Vegetables and Fruit

3 servings per day</td><td>1 serving is:

• ½ cup raw vegetables
• ½ cup cooked vegetables
• ½ cup tomato or vegetable juice
• 1 small fresh fruit
• ½ cup canned fruit (canned in its own juice and drained)
• 1 cup cubed fruit

*Use caution with skin and seeds.
*Dried fruit may be difficult to tolerate.</td></tr>
<tr><td>Breads, Grains, Cereals

2-4 servings per day</td><td>Recommend servings will vary with energy needs:

1 serving is:

• 1 slice of bread
• ½ cup cooked pasta
• 1/3 cup cooked rice
• ¾ cup dry cereal
• 4-6 saltines</td></tr>
<tr><td>Fats*:</td><td>• Avoid fried and deep fried foods.
• Read labels for fat content of foods.
• Limit fat used for cooking.
• Bake, roast, steam, or coil foods.

Fats are found naturally in foods so limit added fat.</td></tr>
</table>

Different People Have Different Energy Needs

Energy and protein needs vary from one person to the next. The amount of food needed varies depending on age, sex, activity and body size. That is why there is a range of servings for each food group.

Exercise

Surgery starts the weight loss process; daily exercise is required for long-term success. The surgery will help you lose weight for the first year without exercise but weight loss is minimized and weight gain is likely.

Key Points to Remember!

- ✓ Choose foods from all the food groups every day.
- ✓ Avoid fast food.
- ✓ Avoid concentrated sweets.
- ✓ Have a goal of eating three meals a day with a maximum of 1 cup per meal.
- ✓ Limit snacking to one snack between meals of fruit or vegetables.
- ✓ Plan your meals.
- ✓ Read food labels.
- ✓ Know your calorie, protein and fat goals.

Tolerance does not determine what you can eat. You must make a conscious decision about what and how much you eat.

Hydration

- ✓ Avoid drinking fluids with meals.
- ✓ Sip on liquids between meals.
- ✓ Other than nonfat or 1% milk, fluids should provide minimal calories.

✓ Limit use of diet sodas as these contain phosphorus which can bind with calcium and lead to decreased bone density.

Recommended Supplements

You must take a daily supplement for the rest of your life.

Recommended:

Multivitamin with iron-1 daily.
Make sure the iron is > 20 mg per pill.

<u>To begin 10-12 months after surgery:</u>
B_{12} – 250 micrograms, 2 per day

Calcium- 1000-1500 mg per day

⇒ Calcium citrate with Vitamin D is the recommended form.
⇒ Start 2-3 months after surgery.
⇒ Take no more than 500 mg at once.
⇒ Do not take at the same time as your multivitamin.

After Gastric Bypass you are at high risk for vitamin and mineral deficiencies over the long term. You may need additional supplements as time passes. Be sure to have your labs done annually (including a CBC, Chem 12, Iron/TIBC, and B_{12}/folate) and take supplements as recommended by your physician or dietitian.

The following sample menus have approximately 1000 calories per day:

Day 1
BREAKFAST
1 poached egg
1 slice wheat toast
1 tsp margarine

SNACK:
1 small apple
1 oz mozzarella cheese

LUNCH
2 oz tuna
1tsp light mayonnaise
Sliced tomato
2 oz pretzels

- 2 cups nonfat milk throughout the day

DINNER
3 oz broiled haddock
1/3 cup green beans
¼ cup white rice

Protein: **73 grams**
Fat: **26 grams**

Day 2

BREAKFAST
½ cup cottage cheese
½ pear

SNACK
6 oz light yogurt

LUNCH
2 oz chicken breast broiled
1/3 cup carrots cooked
1 tsp margarine
¼ cup pasta salad

- 2 cups nonfat milk throughout the day

DINNER
½ cup black beans
¼ cup white rice
1 tbsp salsa
1/3 cup lettuce
½ tbsp Italian dressing

Protein: **70 grams**
Fat: **22 grams**

Day 3
BREAKFAST
¾ cup Cream of Wheat
¼ cup canned pears

SNACK
1 orange
¼ cup cottage cheese

LUNCH
1 cup lettuce
¼ cup garbanzo beans
2 oz cheddar cheese
½ tbsp light ranch dressing

- 2 cup nonfat milk throughout the day

DINNER
2 oz broiled sirloin
1/3 cup mashed potato (made with milk)
1/3 cup asparagus tips

Protein: 62 grams
Fat: 24 grams

Chapter 13

Fitness

In the past, fitness was always the one thing that I gave up on first when I hit my goal weight. I knew going into my Gastric Bypass Surgery, that I not only had to change my eating habits forever, but I would also have to commit to a lifetime of fitness. I knew in my heart that it would take both proper eating and fitness to lose my excess weight. I also knew proper eating and fitness would be necessary to maintain my body weight once the excess weight was gone.

I am not an expert in fitness, and I made several mistakes starting my fitness program after surgery, but I do feel strongly when I say that without a continued fitness program, or fitness activity after your initial weight loss, you are going to be at risk of gaining some or all of your weight back. As you may know, and I have said on a couple of occasions in this book, Gastric Bypass is nothing more than a tool to help an individual lose an excessive amount of weight over a period of one year to 18 months. Without a true commitment to changing your life forever, this includes the other two tools: making the proper food choices and maintaining a proper level of fitness, then Gastric Bypass Surgery will become nothing more than a very expensive failed weight loss program.

So please, read about how I started my fitness program. Learn from my mistakes, and gain from my experience.

When I first researched and consulted about Gastric Bypass Surgery, I read a brochure which said to do 30 minutes of cardio exercise a day, and to do it five days a week. Because I felt I had more weight to lose than the average Gastric Bypass patient, I decided I would exercise 30 minutes a day for seven days a week instead of five. I did not realize this was a mistake, and I will explain later why you do not want to exercise seven days a week.

I still remember my first support group meeting. It was on the 5th floor of the hospital. The elevator only went up to the 4th floor. You had to take a flight of stairs to the 5th floor, and then walk down a long hallway. When I arrived at the meeting at 390 pounds, I sat down in a chair, very much winded and a little sweaty. I overheard two ladies sitting nearby, and apparently midway through their weight-loss journey. They were talking about how nice they felt. One of the ladies exclaimed that she had parked her car down the street, and she had run up all five flights of stairs, and then expressed how great she felt. I said to myself, *"Yeah right,"* and couldn't believe what I had just heard. So I decided to make this one of my first fitness goals. Down deep inside, I wanted to own that statement. So over the next six months of support group meetings, I conquered one flight of stairs at a time, until I too was able to run all five flights of stairs without being overly winded, and I never looked back.

As hard as it is at an extreme weight to even think about exercise, you have to develop a mind set to make the change, to set goals, or it will never happen. As I later found out, everything you do is 90 percent mental, 10 percent physical. Even baby steps are a good start, but you must always challenge yourself to improve. While you are losing your initial weight, you must push yourself every step of the way, and not be satisfied with doing the same thing over and over just to get the exercise component out of the way. You must accept the following clichés: "No pain, no gain;" "Nothing ventured, nothing gained;" "If you don't do it right the first time, you'll just have to do it over again." All three of these clichés are relevant to how I started my fitness program.

Initially I started my own fitness routine on my treadmill at home. I was embarrassed about my size, and I did not want other people to see me while I struggled to do my workout. I did not breathe well during my workouts, and I sweated profusely. I just did not want other people to gawk at the "fat lady" when I was working out. So the home workout was perfect for me. Anyway, gyms are filled with fit and skinny people, so I thought, and I was very intimidated about the machinery in the gym. How would I know how to operate those machines, and for how long? What if I was too heavy for the machines? Would someone tell me not to go on certain machinery, or would they only notice after I broke it?

There was way too much to worry about to join a gym. It will be easier if I did my 30-minute workout at home. So I did.

When I first began my cardio workouts on my treadmill, I was able to walk 2.4 miles an hour. So I was able to walk 1.2 miles in a 30 minute workout. I did this 30-minute workout on a level one, which is a flat level surface. This workout was okay for the first month, but I knew I needed to challenge myself and push to a new goal. I fell back on my past experience with *Body for Life* workouts and broke my workout into six workouts of five minutes each.

I would do my first minute at 2.5 miles an hour, and the second minute at 2.6 miles an hour, and the third minute at 2.7 miles an hour, and fourth minute at 2.8 miles per hour, and finally the fifth minute at 2.9 miles per hour. I would do this for six sets or so.

As I felt comfortable doing this, I would start the baseline at 2.6 miles an hour for one minute and then increase each minute by a tenth of a mile an hour. Each time my sets felt comfortable, I would increase another tenth of a mile an hour for my baseline, and go up from there. I felt like I could do anything one minute at a time. Then an amazing thing happened over the next eight weeks, 2.5 miles an hour actually seemed slow, so by increasing walking speed by one increment at a time, I was able to increase my base from 2.5 miles an hour to 3.0 miles an hour. All done one baby step at a time.

I basically did this cardio workout seven days a week for the first 12 weeks. I did not add any lifting or weights to the workout. But I did add other little fitness-wise things to my daily routine. I started parking my car at the end of the parking lot, so I could have a brisk walk into a store.

In the past, I would circle the parking lot to find the closest parking place to a store, even if this meant circling the parking lot a few extra times. I even went to the extreme of parking in the spaces reserved for those with handicaps. I was a back-up driver for my mother-in-law Maryann, who had HP placards. I deceptively and dishonestly used that placard when I was alone.

I did other positive steps to achieve better fitness. I would walk every aisle in a store whether I needed to go down that aisle or not. I would climb a flight of stairs instead of using the elevator to go up one or two floors. All these little things do add up over time, and help you achieve better health.

Thanksgiving 2004, Dale and I took another seven-day trip to Florida. I desperately wanted to reach the century weight loss mark prior to leaving; however, I was only able to get to a total loss of 96 pounds before we left on vacation. We visited a friend in Daytona and we all went to a gigantic swap meet set in the infield of the Daytona International Speedway 2.5 mile tri-oval. So each time we went down one row, we had walked nearly half a mile. We walked all over that track that day, and I wasn't even tired!

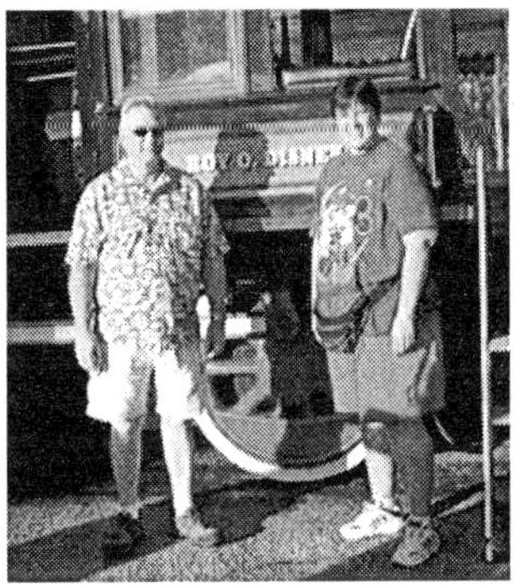

Thanksgiving 2004 – had lost 96 pounds, Weighed 296.

We spent the remaining five days in Disney World where we did a lot of walking. We also asked for a room on the third floor of our hotel, so we could walk the stairs each time we went to and from our room. This was the first time at Disney World that I was able to go on most of the rides without crushing my husband. I actually had room to spare on most rides.

On our way back from Florida, I was reading one of the in-flight magazines, and I saw that Disney World hosted a half marathon on my birthday and a full marathon on the day after. I thought to myself. *It sure would be fun to come and walk the half marathon. I also thought what a great excuse it would be to come back to Disney World.*

Another important milestone on this trip was the bathroom on the plane. This was the first airline flight I had taken since I was a child where I was actually able to fit into the airplane bathroom

Prior to this trip I had been kind of stagnant in my current weight loss. I had only lost a few pounds over the two weeks prior to our vacation, so I was very happy to find out when I got home that I had lost 11 pounds.

In January 2005, I had my six-month check up with my surgeon. At the three-month follow-up, he praised me for my efforts, but for some reason, it seemed he was disappointed with my progress. I was down approximately 125 pounds. I had lost over half of my weight loss goal. But everything from his body language to what he said seemed to me that he was disappointed. He asked, "Sooo have you started your weight training yet?" I had meant to have started lifting by then, but I was just too busy. Between work, home, and my daily cardio workouts, I just didn't seem to have time. So I told the doctor that I had not started lifting; however, I did mention the idea of walking the half marathon the following year at Disney World. He replied in jest with the following: "Maybe you should run the entire marathon."

In retrospect, I know he was just trying to let me know how many options or possibilities were opening up for me as I was losing my weight. He knew if I was 300 pounds lighter, that I could do practically anything I set my mind to physically. However, deep down inside I felt I could do better than I was currently doing for myself regarding my fitness. I recall thinking, *"Just wait, he'll see results!"* Then that marathon statement started to set in. As I left his office, I began thinking, "*Wow! Does he really think I could run a full marathon? He must know something I don't know. Okay, I'll do it!*"

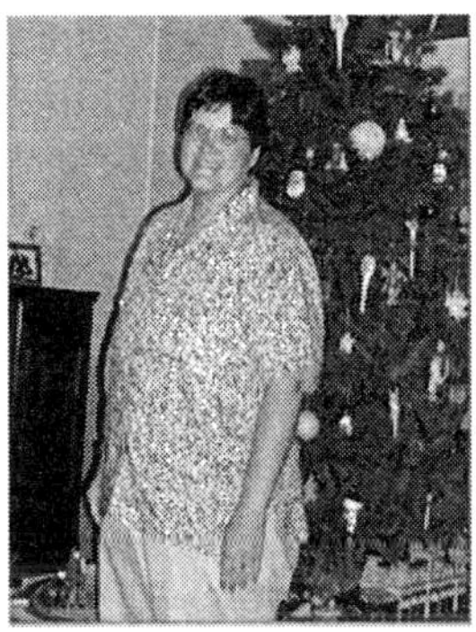

Six months – had lost 125 pounds,
Weighed 267 pounds.

Ironically, at my next support group meeting, a representative from the YMCA came to tell us what kind of fitness programs their gym had. The meeting was very informative. He brought brochures, and talked to us about everything that the "Y" had to offer. They have cardio machines, weightlifting machines, free weights, fitness classes (aerobics, Pilates, spinning, and yoga), an indoor basketball gym, racquetball courts, and a couple of pools.

All of this was offered for a very reasonable membership price with a family discount. We were also informed that financial aid was available for families who needed help.

During this meet and greet, we were all informed that the "Y" offered a quick-start fitness program. You could receive two free sessions with a personal trainer at no additional charge after your initial membership. The way the quick-start program worked was a trainer did a consult with you to find out your fitness goals, and then the trainer would set you up and show you how to do a proper cardio workout. This included showing you how all the cardio machines work. The second session with the personal trainer would be two to four weeks later, and during that session she would help you identify which weight lifting machines you should start using in your workout, and show you how they operate. They also had a brochure for personal trainers with ala carte pricing.

I was very much exited about what I found out about "Y" at the meeting, and I was ready to take my fitness to the next level. I rushed home to let Dale know what I had found out. Dale did not have the same enthusiasm as I did about joining the "Y," so the idea of joining a gym was shelved for awhile.

Over the next couple of months I would look at the brochure I kept for the YMCA. After a slow weight loss of 8 pounds in January and February combined, I decided to give the "Y" a try. I decided to sign up just myself, and add a full 10 sessions with a personal trainer. I planned on spreading out the sessions. So for the first three weeks I went five days a week. Twice a week I worked out with my new trainer, Jolene, at the West "Y" in Boise. I decided to go twice a week for the first three weeks because I wanted some accountability to my new workouts, like I have at my job. If I was to miss a workout, then like my work, my trainer would say, "Hey, where's Anita-Nell?" Also, my first workouts were used to help me get familiar with the machinery, and build form and coordination. As a heavy person, I needed to work on my form and coordination every time I lost about 50 pounds. It's like working out with a whole new body.

I sat down with Jolene in the beginning to let her know my short-term and long-term goals. It was pretty obvious that my short-term goal was to find the right cardio and weight workout to augment my weight loss. And my long-term goal was to build muscle and stamina so I was able to run a full marathon, as my doctor had inspired me to do during my last check-up.

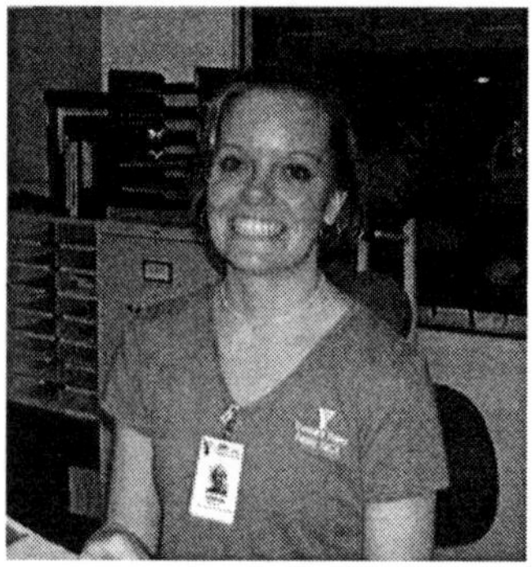

Jolene, my personal trainer.

Jolene, who was a runner in high school and a rower in college, pulled back on my reins for the full marathon. She felt if I entered the full marathon too soon and failed, that my chances of ever entering another would be slim to none. So after going over my initial weight loss and fitness activity since the surgery, she felt it was a very achievable goal not only to enter the half marathon, but to run it as well. She knew she had almost a year to succeed with this goal.

I spent the first three weeks using just the treadmill and some weights seven days a week. I started with weight machines, but as time went on, I did a lot with free weights. I not only learned form and coordination in the first three weeks, but also balance. Jolene had me doing exercises using stretching bands and a BOSU ball to help crest this balance.

I lost 22 pounds in the first 3 weeks. I was so excited about making the decision to join the "Y." I spent the next four weeks going to the "Y" and working out six days a week by myself. One day a week I would work out with my personal trainer. We would work out on the same day every week.

I was still working out seven days a week until another trainer at the "Y" ratted me out to Jolene. She sat me down and told me why working out seven days a week was not beneficial. The biggest reason is that you have to give your body a day of rest to recover. Without that day of rest, your muscles do not have the same opportunity to rejuvenate and grow. Just like weight lifting, you want to alternate different muscle groups, so you do not work out on the same muscle two days in a row. The same holds true with walking or running; however, you then want to rest one to two days after five consecutive days of working out. So she put some big-time boundaries on my workouts. I was not ever to go more than six days in a row, and every three weeks I was to only go five days in a row, and take two days of rest.

After the 10 sessions ended, I felt better than I ever had before doing physical fitness, so I elected to sign up for 10 more sessions. With Jolene by my side once a week, it was easier to push myself to higher levels. Every week she would challenge me little by little during the workouts. She would push me a little harder, or have me try new cardio machines or weight machines.

She would say, “Hey Anita-Nell, have you tried any of the other cardio machines yet? I have to work out on the elliptical machine today, do you want give it a try?” Of course after the first five minutes I was whipped. But I did not want to let her down, so I went the entire 20 minutes. She complimented me, and made me very proud that I was able to do it, and then she continued to run for an additional 20 minutes for her 40 minute workout. I was very impressed. About every 3 weeks, she would use the same line, “Hey Anita-Nell, have you tried this other cardio machine yet? I have to work out on it today, do you want give it a try?” Eventually, I was working out and alternating with every cardio machine. One of the most complete workouts I got came from the rowing machine, and because Jolene was a rower in college, she was able to teach me perfect form. This workout would work every muscle in my body. I used the rowing machine quite often.

I signed up three and a half times with a personal trainer for a total of 35 workouts. My workouts slowly went from walking to jogging to running on all of the cardio machines. So I began to use what is called the 3-2-1 method. It is a pretty simple plan:

I would do the following:

3 minutes walk
2 minutes run
1 minute walk
3 minutes run

2 minutes walk
1 minute run

Then repeat. I would do three sets when I first started.

After practicing the 3-2-1 for a month or so, I dropped the 1 minute and did the following 3-2:

3 minutes walk
2 minutes run
3 minutes walk
2 minutes run

After further time passed, I changed it to 2-3 or 2-4:

2 minutes walk
3 minutes run
2 minutes walk
3 minutes run

You get the idea,

2 minutes walk
4 minutes run
2 minutes walk
4 minutes run

By the middle of June my weight was down to 214 pounds. Jolene thought it was a good idea to take some of the workouts outside in preparation for the half marathon training. The first thing I had to do when switching to outside workouts was to invest in a good pair of orthotics for my shoes. Orthotics is removable shoe inserts that are placed in walking shoes to remedy any discrepancies in the foot position. They enhance shock absorption, weight distribution, and alignment of the feet and body while walking.

For the first two weeks outside we just did some long walks. Around the third week, during our walk Jolene would start to run. Of course I would have to run too. I never knew when we would stop running and go back to walking. At first we would run just 100 yards or so, and then we would return to a walk. But the runs would slowly and gradually get longer and longer. At first I did not like to run. It was very hard work, and I was totally out of my established comfort zone of walking. As we ran, I recall looking on the side of the road or path for a point where I thought we would eventually stop running. Okay, I see a garbage can ahead, a tree, or a water fountain. Maybe we will stop there. I remember saying to myself, *"Just keep going, we are probably going to stop when we get to that tree."* Many times we would just run right by, and I would have to pick a new marker to will myself to continue on. The more walks and runs we did, the easier it became.

As I approached my one year anniversary of the Gastric Bypass Surgery, I was hoping to reach a total of 200 pounds lost. The last pounds are always the hardest to lose. So I worked extra hard, especially at running. At my one year mark, I had lost a total of 198 pounds. I now weighed 194 pounds. Even though I was two pounds short of my goal, I had lost over half my total weight by four pounds. I was very proud of myself.

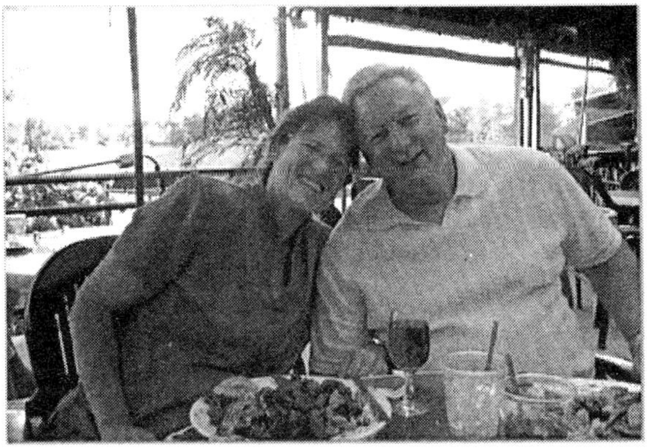

1 year –I had lost 198 pounds, Weighed 194 pounds.

I went to the gym daily, and continued my cardio and weights. I still took off one day a week, and two days off every three weeks. As you may know if you ever have lifted weights, muscle is heavier than fat. So as your muscle builds and becomes larger, there may be a plateau in weight loss, but the larger the muscle, the more calories that muscle burns. So eventually your larger muscles become an asset for you in losing weight, and in keeping the excess weight off.

As time went on, Jolene and I would meet as friends outside the gym to go for a run. I continued to use the 3-2-1 training method to learn how to run further. I ran my first half marathon on my birthday, January 7th, 2006, in Walt Disney World in a time of 2 hours, 25 minutes. I will talk more about this in the running chapter.

At 16 months, I had my body fat tested. I was 12-1/2 pounds from my goal weight. I weighed 174.5 pounds, my lean body mass was 144.1 pounds. This means my body fat was 17.4 percent. For a female from 40-49 years of age anything under 20 percent is considered excellent.

It took six months to lose the last 30 pounds. I pushed myself extra hard in the last six months with my fitness, and I was able to make my goal weight of 162 pounds just four days past the 18-month anniversary of my surgery. My blood panel also came back with great results. Dr. Oakley was amazed at how low my cholesterol numbers were compared to a year earlier. I have now increased my eating slightly and joined a running club. I have maintained my goal weight of 162 pounds for more than a year, and plan on maintaining it for a lifetime.

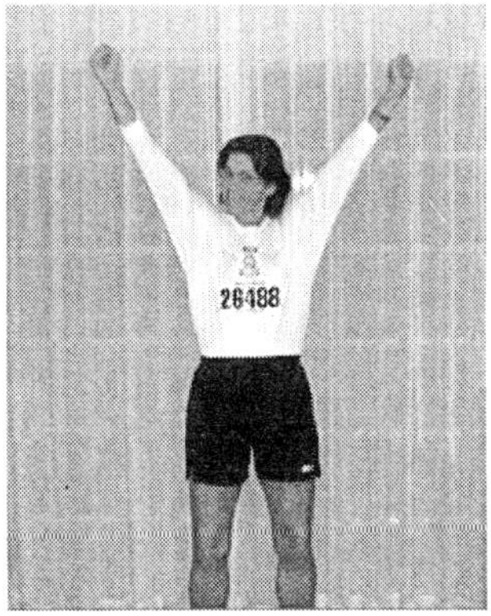

This picture was taken the morning of my first half marathon. (Chapter 16) I was three weeks and five pounds short of my goal weight of 162.

As you can see by reading this chapter; my fitness got off on the wrong foot. No pun intended. I did two major things wrong. I worked out improperly for the first six months because I was working out seven days a week, and not allowing my body to rest. I also waited too long to get the help and advice I needed earlier to properly work out.

So please let me give you just a little advice about proper fitness. Spend the first two weeks getting used to your body, and allow your body to heal from the surgery. Take long walks, either around your neighborhood, at a local school track, or on a treadmill at home. Keep yourself accountable, and walk a little further each day. Do what I finally learned. Work out six days and then relax one day, and every three weeks work out five days in a row and take two days off. Then pat yourself on the back for a job well done!

On your first two days off, start researching gyms in your area. I highly recommend the YMCA, but do not limit yourself, especially if there is not a YMCA close to where you live. The gym has to be convenient. If it is too far away, you will use that later as an excuse to take days off. It needs to be literally down the street. For those who live in rural communities or counties, then you are used to a long drive anyway. But just think of all that land around you to conquer.

I always think of the "Y" as the blue-collar gym for ordinary people. You do NOT see any of the arrogant or phony people at the YMCA. They are people like you and me. If you find you have a "Y" in your town, but in or through a neighborhood where you do not feel safe, then you may want to choose another gym.

Please try any gym you like. I just ended up at the "Y" in Boise, and I love going there for my workouts. I've actually used all the YMCA's in my area. What I am doing on any given day, and where I am before or where I need to go after my workout, determines which facility I use that day. I use the one that is most convenient for me and my schedule on that day.
It is not absolutely necessary to have a personal trainer. However, I feel if you have gone this far in your commitment to change your life, then what is a

little extra money for great fitness advice. The money is spent over time, and not all at once. Besides the great advice, Jolene kept me accountable to my workouts. Trust me; you never want to look a trainer in the eye after a missed workout. We always met on the same day every week, unless I was out of town on business or on a vacation, in which case, we would met the following week on the same day and time. I would always let her know ahead of time if I was going to be out of town, and never used that as an excuse not to work out.

Single and family memberships for the YMCA are very affordable. And as mentioned before in this chapter, all YMCA's have some kind of financial assistance program. They will never turn anyone away. The YMCA is worldwide, and you are able to visit any "Y" in the world at no additional charge. This benefit is included in your membership. So you have no excuse for not working out, even on extended vacations or visits. The great thing about the "Y" is they also offer a variety of fitness classes such as aerobics, spinning, basketball leagues, and softball leagues for adults. These are nice to join after your initial weight loss. They keep you moving and off the couch at home.

If you elect not to use a personal trainer, but decide to join a gym, then make sure you are accountable to yourself. Don't make up excuses, always push yourself to the next level, and always do some level of physical activity, or you will at risk of regaining your weight

My final topic in the fitness chapter is stretching. It is vital as you lose weight that you stretch your muscles as part of your fitness routine. Whether you are doing aerobic exercise, weight lifting or a combination of both, it is very important to stretch your muscles before and after your workouts.

Fitness experts recommend that at a minimum you stretch at the end of your workout to remove extra lactic acid which has built up in your muscles while you were exercising. As the muscles tire, they produce this lactic acid, which is a fuel for the muscle. Lactic acid is what causes the soreness in your muscles. So when you stretch, fresh or new blood travels to that muscle, allowing the muscle to release the built-up lactic acid. You should stretch several different times to circulate the blood.

However, obese people have shorter muscles because of the fat on their body, so stretching before a workout to warm up or loosen the muscles should become an essential part of your workout routine as you lose weight. This can help prevent a pulled or strained muscle during your workout.

To visualize why obese people have shorter muscles, just picture the fat around the arm and shoulder, and how high or far away the arm and/or hand rest away from the side of the body. Therefore, the muscles on the shoulder and arm are shorter than if the fat was not on there. If the fat was not there, then the arm or hand would rest closer to the body, and the muscles would be longer.

Lactic acid also causes a burning sensation if you push your muscles too quickly. Like when you run. If you start running too quickly it could cause your muscles to build up the lactic acid rapidly and cause your muscle to burn. However, if you stretch prior to running and start off slower, your muscle will not hurt because the lactic acid will develop at a much slower rate, which your body will be able to absorb. So you will not feel it as much.

Chapter 14

Support Groups

As outlined in the pre-surgery chapter, it is very important to find a doctor who offers a support group before and after your surgery. This group should meet monthly or bi-monthly.

I attended my first support group meeting two months prior to my surgery. At the time I went to my first meeting, my surgery had not yet been scheduled, nor had I had my initial consult with my surgeon. I actually went to my first support group meeting to gather information about Gastric Bypass Surgery.

The first meeting I went to, I just sat there and observed and listened, and did not say a thing. During this meeting I heard that most patients usually attend around 18 months. Some of the reasons patients stop going are: they become much busier in life, they reach their weight loss goal, or they just do not have time any more for the meetings. Another reason some patients stop going is the embarrassment of weight gain. We were told during this meeting that if a patient ever started gaining weight this was actually the time they needed to attend the meetings for support, and not to stop coming. By removing your support, your chances of permanently going off track are much greater. It is better to surround yourself with people who know what you're going through than to alienate yourself from the group.

I basically attended my support group for the first six months as a resource to my after-surgery life. In these meetings I would find out what kind of foods and vitamins other patients were taking. I would find out if others were dumping the same foods I was, or what exercises the rest of the group was doing. The meetings became a confirmation to me. I was able to judge or gauge my progress by listening and comparing my steps to those in the group. I did more listening than sharing during this time.

One of the most awesome benefits of a support group is a clothing exchange, which our group does three times a year. If your current group does not offer this benefit, then I suggest you organize it. For a clothing exchange, members bring clothes that are too big for them now and members who are now in those sizes can take them home. You don't necessarily have to bring clothes to participate, but it makes for a better selection for others if you do. During the exchange you should gather clothes at least four sizes smaller than your current size, because you will drop at least four sizes between exchanges (unless you're very close to your goal). Buying new clothes every month or couple of months is very expensive, and the exchange will save you a ton of money. Any clothes that remain after the exchange is over are donated to a local women's shelter.

Here is an example of how the exchange works: For work, I am required to wear either black or tan pants. So during each exchange, the first thing I would look for is black or tan pants in my next four sizes. Next I would select one nice outfit for each size, and then look for whatever else I could find. You should always prioritize what your needs are before each exchange because clothes can be chosen quickly once people start looking.

At the next exchange, I would always bring back what I took from the last exchange; and any clothes in my closet that no longer fit. This usually included some new clothes I had purchased. However, I did have a couple dozen expensive business suits that I had purchased over the years in sizes ranging from 26-36. I sold these outfits on eBay over time for about $900.00. I banked this money exclusively for underwear, bras, and workout gear. This $900.00 was completely eaten up buying undergarments when I went from a size 38 to size 8/10.

The support groups are also great for working out emotional issues you may have at home, work, and play. Some of the topics we covered over the last year are relationship changes after weight loss surgery, emotional eating, vitamins and supplementation, importance of protein, exercise, Kettlebells, and learning to walk and run. Besides these topics and great guest speakers for meetings, we would also have complete meetings with open topics or discussion, which allowed us to bring up our own concerns. We always had time at the end of each meeting, regardless of the topic, to bring up questions or other topics for discussion.

I found that over time it has become easier to build friendships from my support group. I have made six very close friends, and what I consider lifelong friends, from my support group. I love them dearly.

Over time, the meetings have also offered me the opportunity to reach out to the newer patients as a mentor. As my life has changed, my main goal is to inspire others. I have now attended the same support group for two and a half years. I think it is very important that support groups have senior or seasoned veterans of the Gastric Bypass Surgery attending. It becomes such an inspiration to the new members to see, visit with, and question the senior members of the group. I consider this my way of giving back. I have come to the conclusion that as long as I am in town, I will always attend my monthly meeting to help others. I also encourage others to attend indefinitely too, as I plan on attending a lifetime. This makes for an unbelievable support group, with long-term ties and a shared history.

Finally, the support group plans Holiday Parties. These are always great for new recipes. We always have a potluck where we are encouraged to make something new and creative to share.

Chapter 15

Commitment and Transfer Addiction

Commitment: com·mit·ment kəˈmɪtmənt – Pronunciation [k*uh*-mit-m*uh*nt] – noun

1. the act of committing.
2. the state of being committed.
3. the act of committing, pledging, or engaging oneself.
4. a pledge or promise; obligation: *We have made a commitment to use all the tools of Gastric Bypass Surgery.*
5. engagement; involvement: *I have a sincere commitment to change my life.*

Gastric Bypass Surgery, as explained before, is not a miracle cure. It is only one tool or one of the prongs in a much bigger weight loss commitment. The surgery should not be taken lightly. It will take a real commitment on your part. No one is going to lose the weight for you and keep it off. You will need to make a real commitment and make several life-changing decisions; the first being that you believe the surgery is one of the necessary tools.

If you make no other decision other than to just have the surgery, then you are going to still lose weight because of the restrictive size of your stomach. But without a further commitment of healthy eating and achieving a minimum level of fitness, you will run the risk of gaining some, if not all, of your weight back.

Normally when we go on a diet, we change our eating habits temporarily, and then once our weight loss goal is reached, we return to our previous bad eating habits, and we regain our weight.

It will take a lifetime commitment to healthy eating once you have the surgery. I remember when I went into my three-month check-up with my surgeon. I had printed a bunch of stuff off the internet about my actual calorie intake. I was super proud of myself when I presented this to my doctor. He looked me square in the eye and said, "Anita-Nell, you are not on a diet. You are learning how to eat as a thin person. When a thin person feels full, they stop eating. Because of your surgery, you now have the opportunity to know what it is like to feel full." That hit me in the head like a ton of bricks, and the magical light bulb finally turned on. It was then that I first realized that the choices I was making then would be the same choices that I needed to make for the rest of my life. It was a decision and commitment on my part to continually eat in a healthy manner, and to know when to stop eating. You too will not be dieting. You will learn to make healthy food choices for the rest of your life, and learn to eat up until, or right before you reach that feeling of fullness. It is a true commitment on your part.

Reflecting back again to my three month check-up, my doctor also said, "You are not only supposed to eat like a thin person, but are supposed to behave like a thin person." He challenged me to observe the way thin people behave. Not all thin people exercise regularly, but most have some type of fitness level they are engaged in. Some play with their kids, some are active in sports or outdoor activities, some take daily or nightly walks, and others work out at their local gym. For the most part, a majority of thin people eat smaller portions, and engage in some level of physical activity.

As you approach your goal weight, you must remember your stomach pouch has enlarged over time, so you will be able to eat larger portions of food. This is why it is vital to continue to be active. You need to reach the point where you actively burn all of the calories your body takes in on a daily basis.

So it is my advice for you to find some level of physical activity that you truly enjoy, and continue to hold yourself accountable to it, so you will do this level of fitness on a daily basis with enjoyment. I really don't care how you do it, you just need to get out there and move! Get your body moving and do something!

Your commitment needs to be 100 percent for all 3 prongs (surgery, eating, and fitness) in order for your weight loss to be successful for life. I hear all the time from people that hear my story, "You are so committed to fitness. You're not the norm!"

This statement is typical, and is why you need to make it a lifetime commitment and not just a temporary change in your lifestyle. If you want to maintain your weight loss, you need to make a true commitment, a lifetime commitment.

Transfer Addiction

Prior to my surgery, I was not given a lot of information about this topic. However, I feel it is important enough that I let you know what I know now.

Addiction is defined in the Word Net dictionary as: "*Being abnormally tolerant to and dependent on something that is psychologically or physically habit-forming.*"

I read somewhere that 90 percent of morbidly obese people are overweight because of an emotional addiction to eating. This means that there is already some kind of underlying psychological or emotional problem that causes morbidly obese people to habitually eat. Having Gastric Bypass Surgery does not address or correct the root cause of this behavior. If you have psychological or emotional issues in your life prior to the surgery, then you are most likely going to have the same problems and issues after the surgery.

If you are morbidly obese from a physical addiction to sugar, then the surgery will temporarily fix that because you will not be able to eat much sugar without vomiting for the first year or so after you have the surgery. So the surgery will help you break the cycle of eating a diet high in sugar.

But what experts fear is that you will take your learned addiction to food, and transfer it to another habit to help deal or cope with your emotional problems in life.

Recently I saw an episode dedicated to this subject on the Oprah Winfrey Show. The show specifically focused on three Gastric Bypass Surgery patients with past or present addictions to alcohol and sex.

One of the brave guests sharing her story on the Oprah Show that day was my camp mate Carnie Wilson. She said she battled an addiction to marijuana prior to her surgery. She lost interest after the surgery, and started drinking alcohol instead. After five years of marriage, she said her husband finally gave her an ultimatum: change her behavior, and stop drinking for awhile before they started trying to have a baby, or he was willing to reconsider their relationship. Carnie said she stopped drinking right then, and she got pregnant with her daughter three weeks later. The good news is she has not had alcohol since.

The second Gastric Bypass guest on the show was still drinking. She was in denial that she is even an alcoholic, even though her own family on the show stated they believe she is one. She was drinking up to 10 beers a night. She said she drank because she liked it, and said she could stop at anytime.

The third guest had lost her excess weight, and for the first time was given attention for her physical looks. She had an extramarital affair because of this attention, and then continued to have sex on different occasions with other strangers. I believe her marriage has since ended, and up until the time of this show, she was still unable to change her sexual behavior.

It has been said that the effect of anything you take orally intensifies its effect after Gastric Bypass Surgery. I am not a doctor, but I will try to give you an example in laymen's terms: Alcohol has to travel though your stomach, then to your small intestine where it is absorbed into your bloodstream. After surgery, the alcohol bypasses a large portion of the stomach and goes directly into your small intestine, where it is absorbed into your bloodstream much faster. Some consider the effects of medication and alcohol to be instantaneous after Gastric Bypass Surgery.

As I was finishing this book, my doctor gave me additional information about alcohol and how it is absorbed after Gastric Bypass Surgery. I thought this would be a good place to insert it for your review:

Doctor's Corner

Alcohol in Gastric Bypass Patients

Recent anecdotal evidence has suggested that patients are more susceptible to alcohol following Gastric Bypass Surgery. A large group of Gastric Bypass patients was queried and nearly 90 percent of them claimed they were more sensitive to alcohol after their Gastric Bypass compared to preoperatively. These findings suggest that Gastric Bypass alters the absorption and/or metabolism of alcohol and increases alcohol sensitivity. In a process known as "first pass gastric alcohol metabolism," an enzyme in the stomach (alcohol dehydrogenase) reduces the blood alcohol level and its effects by about 50 percent. It is the alcohol level in the bloodstream that affects the brain and leads to adverse consequences from alcohol consumption. Therefore, a reduction in the blood alcohol level by the action of the stomach is significant. When the vast majority of the stomach has been bypassed, the blood alcohol level is approximately 50 percent higher. Furthermore, not eating while drinking causes alcohol to be absorbed into the bloodstream though the intestine much faster. Investigative studies have shown that alcohol inhibits the absorption of vitamin B1 and other B complex vitamins as well as vitamin B12 and folate. These are all essential vitamins. Using alcohol; therefore, can reduce the intake of required supplements simply if the patient forgets to take them while under the influence. Secondarily, the absorption of those nutrients is reduced because of the alcohol in one's bloodstream.

It is also very compelling to find that individuals with addictions often transfer those addictions to yet another substance such as alcohol. A recent study presented at the

2006 meeting of the American Society for Bariatric Surgery showed that approximately 14 percent of Gastric Bypass patients have increased alcohol consumption post surgery.

The following suggestions are recommended:

1. Do not drink alcohol during the rapid weight loss period.
2. Remember, small amounts of alcohol can cause intoxication.
3. Do not drive or operate heavy equipment after drinking even a small amount of alcohol.
4. If you plan to drink, also eat.

W. Christian Oakley, M.D.

Addictions are mainly viewed in negative terms. When asked to envision a person with an addiction, many of us think of a person addicted to alcohol or illegal drugs, mainly because of the root word addict. You've heard statements throughout your life like: *"He's addicted to women, alcohol, and fast cars," or "I am addicted to sex, drugs, and rock 'n roll."* There always seems to be something inherently bad about a person's behavior when addictions are associated with them.

You rarely hear addiction mentioned in positive terms, like someone being addicted to helping others, volunteering, mentoring, religion, or fitness. It could be said I am addicted to running and fitness, and that I have transferred my habitual eating habits to staying fit. This may be true, but I actually view this as a positive addiction. I am not being physically or mentally hurt by fitness. And my life is not being ruined because of it.

My only advice to you is that if **you don't** smoke, drink alcohol, or take drugs prior to the surgery, then please do not try any of these after the surgery. Because, according to experts, these are addictive substances, and if you take them, you have a greater chance of becoming addicted to them.

In fact, if you do have an addiction to one or more of the above, then you may want to quit or get help in quitting these addictions prior to surgery. The surgery may actually intensify these addictions. Please consult your doctor about any addictions you may have prior to any surgery.

If your addiction to food or other substances is from psychological or emotional problems, then you must find a way to deal with them, and break your addiction, because those same psychological or emotional problems will still be there after the surgery. Which means you will be at risk for transferring your addictions, or intensifying your current addictions. There is nothing wrong with reaching out for help with any psychological or emotional problem you may be having. There are always professional people who can help.

I suggest you research more information on this subject, so that you are aware of the ramifications surgery can have on addictions. Always use your energy and efforts wisely to achieve something positive, and stay away from any substance or behavior that could be physically or mentally addictive.

Chapter 16

Running Toward My Weight Loss Goal

My entire life I could not stand running. It was probably the last activity in the world I wanted to do. It is pretty obvious from my fitness chapter that I avoided the running as part of my fitness routine until the day I declared to my doctor and the world that I was thinking of walking a half marathon. Everything changed from that moment forward. As you may recall from the fitness chapter, my doctor wanted me to realize my full potential after my weight loss, so he suggested that I run the full marathon. When I first approached my personal trainer with this full marathon idea, she thought running was good, but only if I ran a half marathon. I explained her reasons in the previous fitness chapter.

So here I was. I wanted to reach the goal of running the half marathon at Walt Disney World, so the running and training began. Oh man, was it hard to run at first, but I did not take the easy way out, so I actually taught myself how to love running.

13th Annual St. Luke's 5K Women's Fitness Celebration

My very first race was in September of 2005. It was a 5K Women's Fitness Celebration sponsored by St. Luke's Hospital in Boise. I had been training with Jolene for the half marathon coming up in

January. She thought it would be good to run and walk the 5K for my first practice race. To enter the official timed section of the 5K, you had to be able to finish in less than 35 minutes. Because we were running and walking, Jolene didn't feel we could finish the race in that time, so we entered the race as non-timed competitors. During the 5K race Jolene coached me on how to move back and forth and around other competitors as you run. This proved to be very important later when I ran my first half marathon. Up until this point in my training this was the most I had run in a short duration of time. We ended up finishing the 5K unofficially at 33:33. That day I realized the power of my belief, and the incredible strength that always had been there under my weight.

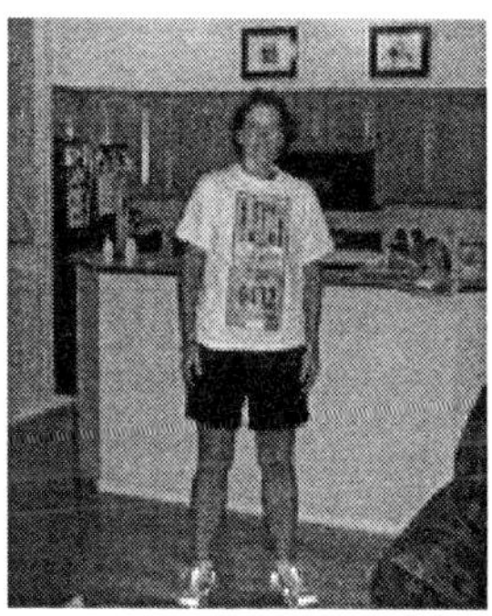

My first 5k run-walk,
St. Luke's 5K Women's Fitness Celebration.

People always ask me, "So when did you run your first mile." It's always hard to pinpoint exactly when I ran a full mile straight; however, I do know when I ran my first two miles consecutively.

I was approximately six weeks away from my first half marathon, and I had not yet run my first consecutive mile. This meant running a complete mile without stopping. Yes, I had graduated from the 3-2-1 system that was explained in the fitness chapter, but now I was walking the first two minutes of every mile I ran. So no matter how many miles I had to run on a given day, I would walk the first two minutes of every mile.

For example: On mile one, I would walk two minutes, and then run out the rest of mile one, and then on mile two I would walk again for two minutes, and then run out the rest of mile two, and so on. So I had not yet run for a complete mile.

The first time I actually ran more than a mile consecutively was on a business trip to Las Vegas. This was the first trip that I had taken while in training for the half marathon. In my training, I had a planned running schedule. My first day in Las Vegas, I needed to walk and run approximately six miles. This was my scheduled workout. As it turned, out the hotel gym was approximately half a mile from my room. I was super pinched for time. I was looking at my watch while I was walking the first mile. I was trying to calculate exactly how much time it was going to take me to go the full six miles while walking the first two minutes of every mile. I did not think I was going to make it. I started to run out the first mile, and then just decided to keep going. I had to; I just did not have the time available for this workout, and I had to get the six miles done. So I ran right into mile number two, and then just kept going from there. I ended up running the full six miles minus the two minutes I walked to warm up. So I guess November 30, 2005, in Las Vegas is the correct answer. Needless to say, my life, and the way I ran and worked out changed one more time as I went to the next level of running.

From this day forward I approached my workouts as a consecutive running workout. No matter how many miles I had scheduled to run, I would walk the first two minutes as a warm up, and then I would run the scheduled miles, and then finally, I would walk five minutes to cool down after I reached the planned miles.

My last scheduled long run prior to my first half marathon was on Christmas Eve 2005. Dale and I were visiting my stepdaughter Kristen and her family in their new house in Seattle. No one was home except Dale and I, and it was our responsibility to assemble a bicycle to go under the tree Christmas morning for our granddaughter Karlee. Kristen and her husband John had set up a treadmill in the garage for me to use for my workouts while I was there. The treadmill was surrounded by boxes that had not yet been unpacked in the move. Dale joined me in the garage for my workout. While I ran, he assembled Karlee's bike. This was the first time that I ran for 2 hours and 20 minutes straight. I ran for 12-½ miles without stopping. It was also the most boring run I had ever done up until this point! I did not have my MP3 player; I was surrounded by boxes, and staring at a garage wall in front of me. Dale was behind me, very much focused on his project, and did not have much to say to me while I ran. I ended up not running the entire 13 miles that night, because of something Jolene had said to me. She said; "Make sure the first time you run 13 straight miles is on the day of the half marathon; that way you will cherish the accomplishment more." As it turned out, it took Dale the exact same time to assemble that little kid's bike. The bummer was we bought the bike fully assembled in Idaho, but since we shipped it to the Seattle area, we had to take it apart and then reassemble it before Christmas.

Walt Disney World Half Marathon

Dale and I arrived in Florida on January 4th, 2006. We spent the first couple of days in Disney World. At the end of the second day, we went to the Disney Wide World of Sports Complex to pick up my official number and race package. When I first arrived, I looked around to see hundreds of buses and thousands of runners getting off them. I said to myself, "*What did I get myself into? I'm just a little amateur runner amongst all these other professional runners*". I started to have a small panic attack, and started to think I was in way over my head. At the same time I had to compose myself. I mean, what was I supposed to say to Dale at that moment, "*Dale, I think I made a mistake, I'm going to withdraw, sorry about all the money we spent getting here".*

Then in my head I could hear Jolene say, *"Anita-Nell, get in your mental game. Running marathons is 90 percent mental and 10 percent physical."* If she was here, she would say, *"You've earned the right to be here. You've done all the physical training; you've lost all the weight. Now you need to stop worrying, and just run the race".* With these thoughts in mind, I became comforted, and thought, *"Yes I can do this."* And my anxiety faded away.

My confidence became stronger once I lined up inside to receive my running packet. While in line, I found that this was the first half marathon for many other runners as well. So my anxiousness subsided further, and I felt even more self assured. After I got my number and running packet, I spent the rest of the day floating on air. It was a very euphoric feeling knowing that I trained all year for this, and I was now less than 36 hours away from my first half marathon.

The following day I went to the running expo with my Disney pals Malinda and Lori, who were also run/walking the half marathon for the first time. My only regret of the entire trip was at the expo. A man behind one of the booths said to me, "So you're a runner?" I actually answered and said, "No, I am a newbie." And the man replied, "Oh, you look like a runner to me." I felt so stupid. *Why didn't I just tell him I was a runner? I was there to run the half marathon wasn't I?* Even to this day, I am mad that I didn't tell him I was a runner. So I make sure to remind people just starting to run that they too are athletes, and they should never discount that fact.

One of the most positive experiences of the expo was meeting with the staff, and then subscribing to *Her Sports + Fitness Magazine*. I have now subscribed for a year, and I highly recommend it. This magazine has no fluff. There is no annoying supplement or diet advertisements in the magazine. They do not use models, all articles are about real people, and they are very inspirational. They have a section called "Women Can Move," where women can send in their own inspirational fitness stories.

Other sections include:

> "Body + Mind,"
> "Fit Foods,"
> "Her Gear,"
> "Discoveries,"
> "Weekend Warrior," and
> "Her Story."

This magazine is the greatest! You can subscribe by going to www.hersports.com.

I also attended a seminar at the expo given by John Bingham, aka "The Penguin" from *Runner's World Magazine*. He is a very slow runner, and looks like a wobbling penguin when he runs. He calls himself a back of the packer, and suggested that you too take your time when running the Disney half marathon, and to soak it all in. You need to get your money's worth, bring a camera, visit the characters, and just enjoy yourself. He was letting the new runners know that it was okay to be in the back of the pack. This was great to hear, and he helped ease our nerves on what to expect. His first book called *The Courage to Start* was a great read, and I only wish I had read it before I started running. So I recommend you read this and his other books when you get a chance.

The alarm clock went off at 2:00 a.m. on my birthday. I was getting ready for my first big race. I took a quick shower, ate a bagel smothered with peanut butter, grabbed a cup of coffee, which I poured into an empty water bottle, and I headed to the bus stop. It was a brisk 32 degrees. Thank God I had the coffee to keep my hands warm. When I arrived at the bus stop, there was only one other runner there. I guess I got there a little early. I had the first-time jitters, and did not want to be late. Malinda and the rest of the runners arrived over the next half hour. We all took buses to the staging area for the marathon.

I was a little worried about Malinda doing the marathon by herself. You see, I was gong to run the half marathon, and Malinda was going to walk and run. So we were not going to be together. She also had not trained as long as I, so I was a little worried about her going the distance. We met a person on the bus who was a fast walker, and who was also alone. Malinda was able to hook up with her for the race. This was great for Malinda because she could pace this fast walker during the race. She would pull ahead of Malinda, and then Malinda would run for awhile and pass her, and then as Malinda started to walk, this lady would again pass her. They did this all through the race.

As I checked in, I looked around at all the other runners jumping around and stretching, and trying to keep warm. It was such a natural high to see all the old and new runners together. Everyone was ready to go. It was so cold. We found a spot where we could huddle around each other to keep warm. We started telling our stories about how we all got there. It was super cool. What a way to start off the morning, it was kind of like camp. Then someone came through and yelled, "Ok it's time to go to your corral."

When you register for a half marathon, you turn in your projected time and then they group you based on your projected time. They call these groups corrals. We got to the staging area about 4:00 a.m., and then about 4:45 a.m., we had to walk about a mile to our specific corral located in the Epcot parking area. For the next hour I watched a pre-run warm-up on the many huge screens to the side of the course. There were different guest speakers, including Mickey and Minnie.

When I signed up nine months earlier, I planned on walking and running the course (like Malinda), so I entered a projected time of 3 hours and 20 minutes. This time put me in the "F" corral, which seemed to be about half a mile behind the starting line. But because of my great training I was now going to run the entire half marathon, and my projected time was 2-½ hours. So I was really in the wrong corral for my running pace. Another runner on the bus told me that when they drop the ropes just prior to the start that I should start jogging up the far left side, and try to get to the runners who would be running my pace. Right about the time I caught up to the group I needed to pace, I crossed the starting line.

I was so pumped up. My first goal was to get to Main Street in the Magic Kingdom. That's where Dale and my support group were waiting for me. It was 5-½ miles from the starting line. As I approached my group, I received a very nice birthday hug and kiss from Dale. It was a quick stop, but I was totally rejuvenated from this encouragement. As I ran down Main Street, I was in awe of the Walt and Mickey statues and the castle in the background. It was like my own private party with the park open only to runners and their supporters.

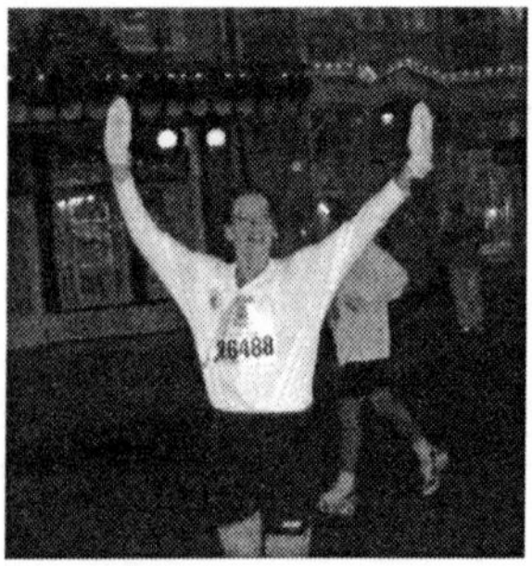

Running down Main Street and floating on air.

As I rounded the corner to Tomorrowland, I rushed into the bathroom for a quick pit stop. No waiting as I went in, but a huge line had formed on my way out. I thought to myself as I was ready to return the course: *"Do you wash your hands or not?"* The debate in my head was not long; I decided to wash them. It was so cool zigzagging through the park as I was running. My picture was taken by a Disney photographer when we left the castle. I exited the theme park through the back staging area of the park. And we ran through this back lot area, we were handed bananas, chocolate, oranges, sports drinks, or water. We just grabbed what we needed. I grabbed bananas and water.

Then I headed back to Epcot to the finish line. As we approached, more pictures were taken. When I got to the 13-mile mark, I just laid it out, and gave it everything I had to the finish line. It felt really good to finish strong.

As we crossed the finish line, we were instructed to enter these shoots, or tunnels. These brought us to an area were our timing chip was removed. The only bummer was our family and friends were left at the finish line and were not allowed back in this area. Once the timing chip was removed, we were given our medals and foil blankets to wrap around us as we cooled downed. Then we got in a long line to have our pictures taken wearing our medals, against a Disney background. I was not able to publish these pictures.

There was plenty of water, sports drinks, and food waiting for us in another area. The whole process took about an hour.

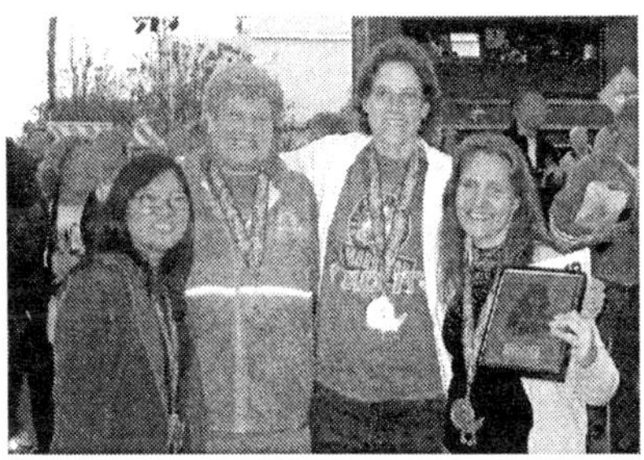

Lori, Malinda, Me, and Debbie

I met Dale, Malinda, her husband Hami, Lori, and my friend Dana after all the post race activities. We recapped how we all did during the race, and what the experience was like for us. We all went out to breakfast. It is amazing how good food tastes after you "give it your all" in a race. After breakfast Dale and I spent the rest of the day at the Magic Kingdom. Malinda and I wore our medals everywhere for the rest of the day. At the end of the day we went to Disney's Famous Boardwalk Bakery, and picked up my sugar-free birthday cake that we had ordered earlier in the week. Dale and I went back to Malinda's Disney timeshare apartment, and we celebrated my birthday with our friends. After the party, we headed to Downtown Disney to the awards ceremony at Pleasure Island. It's amazing that out of 16,000 runners, one of my Disney pals from England ended up winning third place in her age category! Way to go, Debbie!

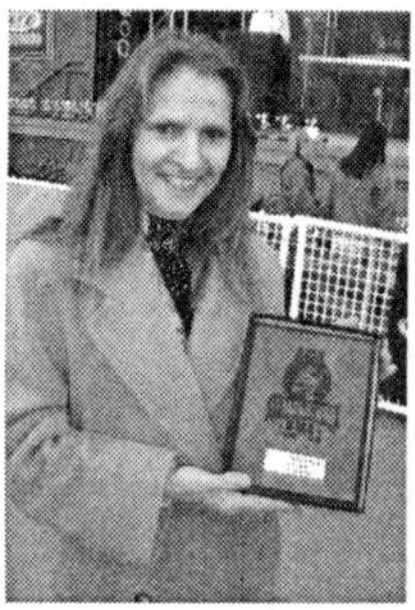 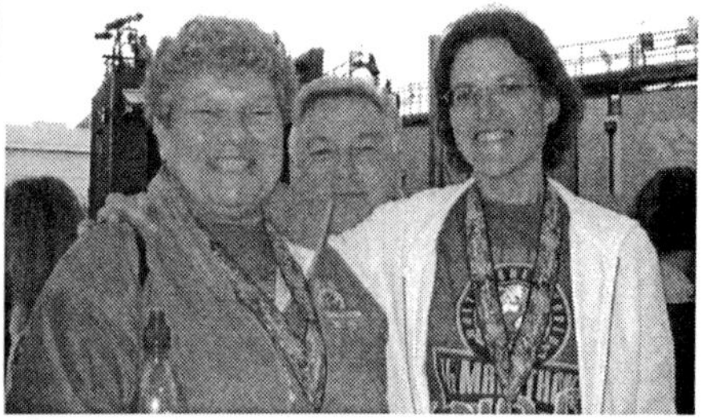

Left: Debbie with third place plaque
Right: Malinda, Dale, and Me with our medals

Running the Disney half marathon was just a fitness goal. When I originally thought about walking and then running the half marathon, I was making the goal as encouragement to losing weight. I thought it would be a nice birthday present to myself after a year and a half of losing weight. But running was how I achieved that goal. When I first made the goal, I thought I would be so fit that I would actually be able to just run it. I didn't think about the training involved, or the actual running I would have to do prior to the marathon to prepare for it. In the beginning I was just focusing on the weight loss. Remember, I did not like running. As a matter of fact, I hated it. Wow, how everything had changed over the past 10 months or so. I actually came to enjoy running, and after I completed the half marathon, I was not sure how I would continue running. But I knew that running had changed my life for ever.

Let's back up just a bit……Prior to the Disney half marathon, I was talking to Stacy at the YMCA. She felt I was doing so well in my run training for the half marathon; she extended an invitation for me to join her BoiseRunWalk.com Club. The club was starting its new year of running events the same day as my half marathon, so if I joined, I would miss the first 2 weeks of running. I asked the director, Steve, if I could come out after the first two weeks and try out the club for a week before I committed. He said that would be fine. The reason I wanted to try it out was two fold. The annual membership was close to $200, and if I joined I would have to commit to running for a least another year. I loved running, but the question was if I wanted to continue running as a sport, or just do it as part of my fitness at the gym? It did not take long to answer that question.

Chapter 17

Running the Extra Mile

This running chapter is the longest chapter in the book. As you read it, you will see how much running has become a part of my daily life, so I felt it was important to pass on my running experience to you. I know many of you will elect not to run or run long distance as part of your fitness activity to aid your weight loss. However, still read forward, because there are some amazing stories ahead. Many of the people in my weight loss support group were not runners prior to meeting me, and now they are not only runners, but they are also inspiring others to run and stay fit. Read on, and see how running has helped me in my weight loss journey.

After I returned from my half marathon at Disney World, I turned my attention to the BoiseRunWalk Club. I felt this was the perfect opportunity to continue my learning about fitness, and it would also keep me accountable to my routine. The club not only ran once a week, but it also had weekly seminars on running and walking techniques, hydration, stretching, recovery, nutrition, and many other topics. However, I would have to make personal sacrifices to join. For the last 20 years I have always worked an early Saturday morning shift, and spent my evenings with Dale. The club met on Saturday morning. So joining the club meant I would have to adjust my work schedule. This meant that I would be getting home after 8 p.m. on

Saturdays. So Dale and I talked about how this would affect our night together. Dale's opinion was that if I joined, I should give it my all, and not worry about our Saturday nights. He felt we had all day Sunday to spend with each other, and we could do something special.

So I joined. The club was a great reinforcement to what Jolene had already started teaching me, and every week I learned something new. But there was a very brief moment when I thought about not joining the club. It was the first week that I gave the club a try. When I arrived at the meeting it was bitter cold and snowing. I thought to myself, *"Okay we will have our meeting, and then go home."* But when the meeting wrapped up, Steve said, "Okay, let's stretch out for our run." I thought to myself, *"Oh crap, he's got to be kidding; they're going to run in the snow. Alrighty then, I'll just slip into my car, and never come back, and I'll tell Stacy later that the running club just wasn't for me."* Then I thought how much I actually enjoyed running, so I agreed to give it a try. I started my stretches.

It was the first time I had run in the snow. It was coming down in big flakes and was absolutely amazing. It was so quiet. There was no background noise, just my own breathing and the squeak of my shoes as I ran through the snow. I was pretty overwhelmed with how peaceful it was. Okay, the first time was great, but it either snowed or there was snow on the ground for the next 10 weeks. When it snowed in Boise, it only seemed to snow on Saturdays when we met, and at no other time during the week. It ended up being a true challenge to go out in the weather every week and run.

Race to Robie Creek

The first big race of the year for the running club is the Race to Robie Creek. It is a half marathon, but because it goes up and over a mountain summit, and a majority of it is on mountain trails, it is just as hard on your body as a full marathon. Every year you can register for the Race to Robie Creek online on President's Day at 8:00 a.m., and by 8:05 a.m. it is full, with 2400 runners.

Up until the Race to Robie Creek most of my running had been on flat land. When I joined the running club, we would run hills every other week. My second week at the running club, we did my first hill run. It was 3 miles uphill, and then 3 miles back. We worked out on the same course the race would be on, so we could prepare for the actual race. Every other week we would increase the distance in preparation for this race. Four weeks prior to the race I pulled my calf muscle. My physical therapist, Matt, who promised I would make the race injury-free, had me do my weekday runs in the deep end of the pool at the "Y." He also had me stretching seven days a week, and doing augmented soft tissue mobilization (ASTYM) treatment twice a week. He allowed me to do one long run on the weekends at an easy pace. You can find more information on the non-evasive ASTYM treatment by going directly to their website: http://www.astym.com/patients.htm.

On the final practice run two weeks prior to the race, we ran 8 miles up to the summit, where we encountered complete white out, and then 4 miles back. As we got within a fourth of a mile of our ride down the mountain, it began to hail. Someone did not want us on the mountain that day.

The day of the Race to Robie Creek I was a little nervous because of my injury four weeks earlier, and all the snow we had over the past two months. But it was a beautiful day. The sun was out, it was clear, and the snow on the ground had melted.

Before the race, Hanna, a woman from the running club, asked if I would run with her. During our practice runs Hanna ran the same or a similar pace as I, so she thought we should run together for timing and support. The race started mid-morning, and Hanna and I took off running together at the same pace. When we got about 2 miles up the hill, as with my first two races, I had to stop and go to the bathroom. When I returned to the course Hanna was gone. So I continued the run by myself up the hill. The run up until this point was fairly easy and very familiar. We had already practiced this hill run for several weeks prior to the race. However, once I got to the summit and headed down the back side, the race became much harder. During practice we only ran up the front side, and then turned around and ran back to the vehicles we drove to the course, so we never got to see the back side during practice.

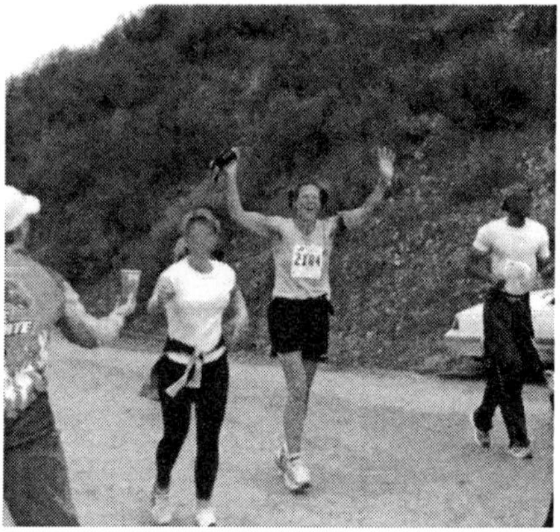

I felt great going up the front side of the course, but was worried while running down the backside.

So I was running alone, and still saw no sign of Hanna. As I went down the backside, I frequently lost my footing in the mud on the steep switchback turns. The ground was very unstable and wet from all the snow we had received over the winter. I did not want to step near the edge of any of the trails, because if the ground gave way, I could fall down the hill. The downhill was so steep that they had to park several vehicles at the apex of the turn to prevent someone from running off the turn and down a cliff.

I spent a lot of time focusing on where to put each step to avoid slipping and injuring myself. Not only was I watching for potholes and loose ground, but for animals that might dart across the course. It was very hard on my knees and legs. I was not sure if I had the stamina to make it. Right around mile 11, I started to become desperate in my thoughts. I was ready to stop running, and just walk. I began to pray to God for the strength to continue. I was asking him just to get me through the remaining 2-½ miles of the race. No sooner had I finished my prayer, I got a tap on my shoulder, and Hanna came running by me. God had answered my prayers. I was so excited to see her. I guess I had passed her somewhere else on the course and did not notice. Maybe she stopped to go to the bathroom? I don't know, and never asked. I do know that I found a whole new strength from within. Hanna and I ran side by side the rest of the way in. We even sprinted together and gave it all we had in the last quarter mile to the finish line. Thank you, Lord! The sign at the fish line said, "LAY DOWN PLAY DEAD." I was ready to do that 2-½ miles back in the race.

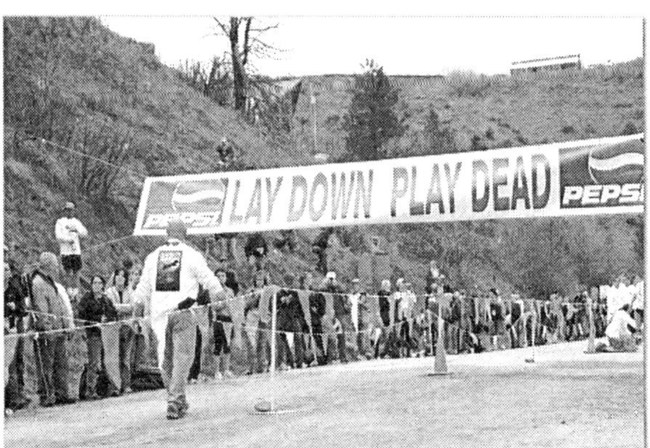

Finish line at Robie Creek.

The post-race activities were very festive. They had loud music playing and a couple of large barbeques going for all the race families and friends. It made for a great post-race atmosphere. To me this race was a mark in my life I will never forget. I felt great at the end of the race. I had a moment where I realized my life had just changed forever once again. Running is a sport where you can be close to God and nature, and you can run alongside your friends, or even strangers, and help each other along. Everyone was running for different reasons and causes, but we all ran because we believed in something. From this day forward I decided I wanted to be able to pass it forward and to inspire others not only to lose weight but to be fit.

Minnie Marathon

The first weekend in May I returned to Florida with my friend Amy to run the Minnie Marathon, which was held during the Weekend for Women, sponsored by the American Heart Association. The actual race was called Run for the Red. Amy is a Gastric Bypass patient and friend from my support group meetings. We had our surgeries just a couple of weeks apart. We found the one great passion we had in common is that we both loved Disney. So during one of our meetings, I had asked if she wanted to go to Walt Disney World with me and enter a 5K and 15K race. She agreed to come and walk it, and I decided to run it. We both attended the running expo on Friday. On Saturday I ran the 5K in a Minnie dress.

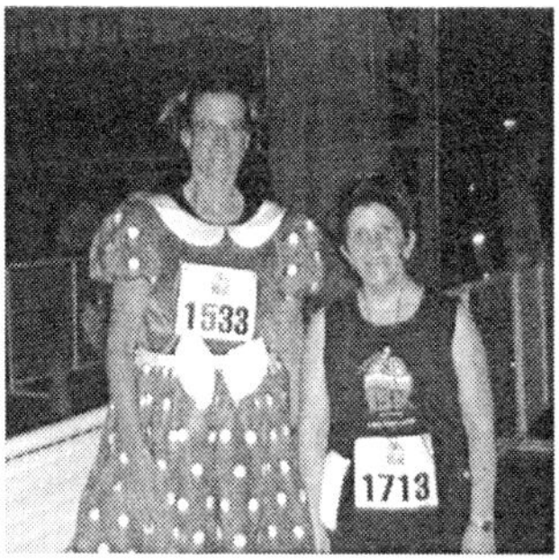

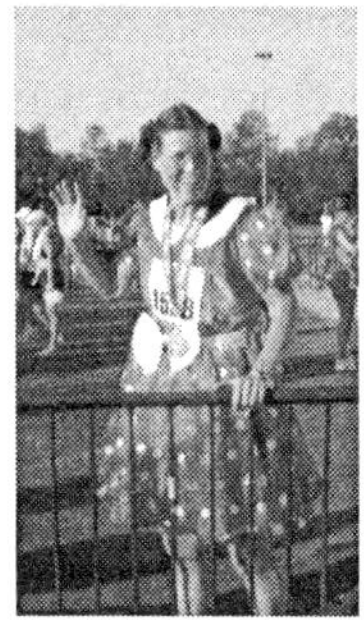

Amy and I - left. The dress made it a little hot, but it was fun!

I came in 10th overall in my age group and 109th overall, with an average time of 9:27 miles. On Sunday, I ran the 15K, and I placed 485th overall with an average time of 10:22 miles. The cool thing was I got to see Amy cross the finish line in tears. She was absolutely on fire emotionally. After the race, she said she finally believed in herself, and felt she could conquer the world. I was so happy for her, and knew exactly how she felt. Since then, Amy has raced a couple of local races on her own, and a couple with me.

5K Race for the Cure

The following week I entered a 5K Race for the Cure, which is the cancer awareness run. I originally was going to run this race, but I had two friends from my support group, Machelle and Linda, who entered this 5K as walkers. I asked them if I could join them, and they said that was fine, but they were only walking, and not going to run. This was good for me because I had run all out the weekend before. I was ready to just enjoy my friends on their first race. Because Machelle's company was one of the major sponsors, all three of us were able to go to a private pre-race breakfast. After breakfast we headed to the starting line early and began to stretch. Before we knew it thousands of people began to line up behind us. Instead of moving back in the pack to where the walkers were, I asked if they wanted to start the race in a run just to make it to the side of the road to let the runners all pass. Then we would walk. They agreed, and said they would run just the start just to get to the side. I also said, "No matter the pace that we walk, we must all three sprint the last 150 feet to the finish line." Again, they both agreed.

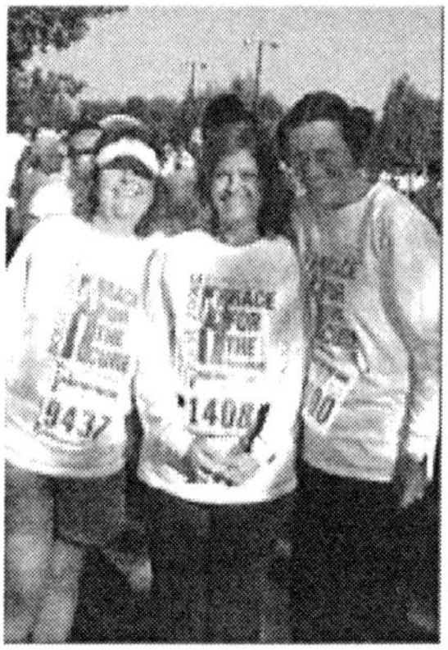

Linda, Machelle, and me.

Once the race started, we all ran to the side, and then ran about a block or so before we slowed to a walk. After a few minutes, Linda said, "Can we start running again?" I said to them, "Are you sure?" They both said yes, so we started running again. I would say, "Okay, we will start to run at the sign and then walk again when we get up to that stop light." We ended up doing this for the entire race. Even though Machelle and Linda had no intention of run-walking the 5K, they did because they were so caught up in the atmosphere of the race. All three of us sprinted to the finish line. My friends were so pumped up; their confidence had jumped to whole new level. They entered the race as walkers with an average pace of 20 minutes per mile. During the race they had increased that average to 15 minutes mile. I was really happy to be a part of that race with Linda and Machelle.

Prior to the Race for the Cure, I had heard about a long race called the Sawtooth Relay in the second week of June. This is a 62-mile relay split between six runners. I was asked to join a relay team by another member at the "Y." However, after my initial invite, I did not hear anything back for a long while. At my April support group meeting I asked if there were any members that would be interested. Six stepped forward, one being Machelle. Linda said she would happy to be an alternate.

Famous Idaho Potato Race

The last race in May was the Famous Idaho Potato Race which was a half and full marathon together. I had entered this race as a runner. This would be the first race I did without a friend. It was a day I will never forget…at least what I can remember!

While standing at the starting line, I did not feel right. I wasn't sure why, but I thought to myself, "*I just need make it through the next two and a half hours.*" Little did I know that after having gone to a celebration dinner on Thursday, I would be one of many (43) to have salmonella poisoning. I progressively got sicker over the first 3 miles. I thought it was the flu, and I could just push through it. I did some running, and then I did some walking. I was still feeling very ill.

I began to stop at every portable restroom along the route. I either had the runs or dry heaved in every one of them. I began to pray for God's help. Soon all I could do was walk. I felt alone, but I knew God was with me. I knew he would pull me through. At mile 12, our friend and coach Steve from BoiseRunWalk Club asked me if I was all right. I explained I thought I had the flu. He asked me if I wanted to stop, and I said, "No, I can go the last mile." By this point I was so out of it, I don't remember how I found the end of the race. It took me 35 minutes to walk the last mile and find the finish line. I am sure I made some wrong turns somewhere, but I finally made it.

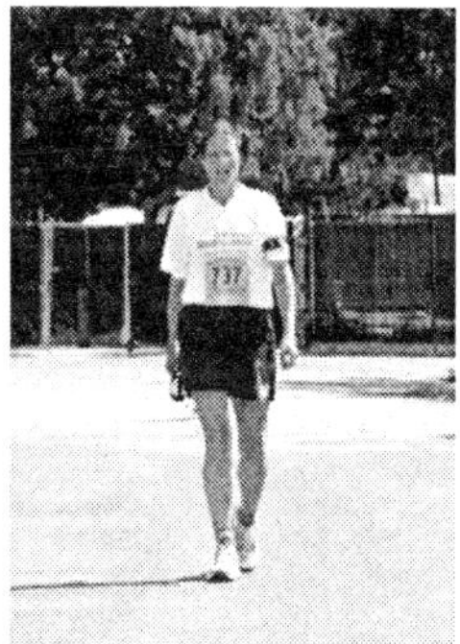

In a dazed and confused walk to the finish line. (IdahoSportsPics)

Two lessons learned. First, when your body is talking to you, it is time to listen. Do not try to be a hero to yourself or others. There is always another race, and always another day to run that race. You do not need to jeopardize your health to prove anything. How lucky I was, considering salmonella can kill you. And here I went ahead and aggravated the poison even further by running 13 miles! Yes, I guess I do have a guardian angel.

The second lessoned learned is not to bunch your races together. I tried to run four races in five weeks or five races in seven weeks if you include the next race, the Sawtooth Relay. As a runner, you need to give your body time to rest and recover. You need to pick and choose your "A", "B", and "C" races carefully. Your "A" races are the long runs, or the events that are most important to you. In these races you are trying to improve on your personal best. These are the events that take up most of your training. You should schedule these races every other month or two months apart. In between the "A" races, you can sprinkle a couple of "B" and "C" races. A "B" race would be more for training, and not an attempt to better a personal time. Instead these would be races you run as a mentor to others. Finally, a "C" race would be events where you walk with someone just starting out. Trust me when I say, you'll be better off scheduling your runs in this manner.

Sawtooth Relay

The next race on the calendar was the Sawtooth Relay. As it turned out, Linda was not able to make this race as an alternate because of a family commitment. This was the first race where I was the chief organizer. It was up to me to get the team members together. I was the one who had to attend the team leader meetings for our group. There were quite a few other responsibilities that went along with being the team leader. I had to recruit a volunteer to help work the relay course, find a place for us all to sleep the night before the relay, make sure we all had the proper gear for the relay, arrange our transportation, and find sponsors for the race who would provide us with shirts, shorts and socks. I also had to lead our group meetings. So basically I was responsible not just for myself, but for our entire group.

Back when I put the group together, Machelle thought I was talking about a local relay, and committed to being one of the six. She had no idea

I was speaking of a 62-mile relay in the Sawtooth Mountains of Idaho. She was pretty floored when she went to the official race website. She came to me concerned that she was too slow because she was only a walker. I told her we were not in the race to win, but to finish. Time was not a factor, just her participation.

On the morning of June 9th we met to decorate our van before we left town for the race. We put our team name "Going, Going, Gone" on the back window. We taped our "before" pictures to the side of the van and wrote how much we had lost next to our pictures. Under our team name on the back window we put 977 pounds, the total weight we had lost.

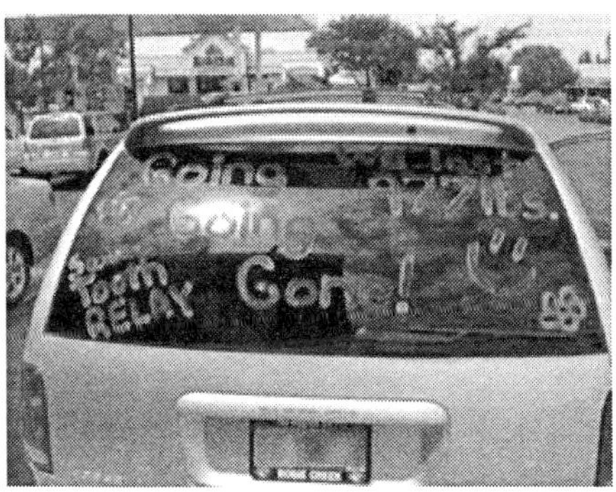

The decorated van we drove to the Sawtooth Relay.

We all had matching shirts with our sponsor's name (Pulse Fitness) on the front, and on the back of each shirt we wrote the following question and answer. The question was: "What Motivates You to Move?"

The answers for the team members were as follows:

Anita-Nell - *To inspire others, and because I can.*
Jen – *Testing my limits.*
Machelle - *My weight loss.*
Tammy - *Going from a size 22 to size 4.*
Amy – *"Goals" and for Nathan & Scotland.*
Carol - *Zoellner Boys, Ryan, Alex, & Sean*

Honorary Members:

Heidi - *Bed sores.*
Carrie- *My hubby in Korea.*

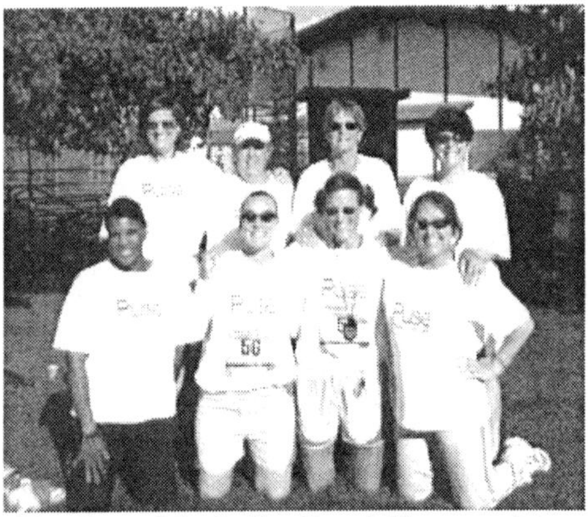

Top Row: Machelle, Carol, Tammy, Amy.
Bottom Row: Carrie, Jen, Anita-Nell, Heidi.
Our team shirts wear sponsored by Pulse Fitness and Running Shop. Meridian Idaho

We set out on our three-hour journey to Ketchum, Idaho. Ketchum was where the finish line was, so we drove the course backwards to the starting line, which was in Stanley, Idaho. On this drive, we were able to see the different segments of the course, and how those segments were rated. As we drove deep into the mountains, nobody expressed it, but we were each a little worried deep inside about our part of the relay. When we arrived at the starting line, we got out and took some pictures. We checked into our hotel rooms, and barbequed our dinner on the deck of the hotel. We had to check in at the starting line by 1:00 a.m. the next morning, so we were in bed by 7:30 that night.

Three of us got a quick night's sleep, and arrived at the race on time. We signed in, and got our race packet. The other three remained at the hotel and sleep thru the night. They would join us later on the course. I was the first leg, so I began to stretch.

Once the race began, and all the runners were on their way, the rest of the team drove ahead to the first exchange point. The first leg was awesome! At the beginning of the race it was pitch black, and for the first three segments of the race, we had to wear head lamps and reflective vests. It was kind of strange. Because it was so dark, you did not have a sense of your speed or distance. I ran on gravel and pavement through Stanley, and then on two different highways. If it had been light, I would have had a full view of the Sawtooth Mountains and the Salmon River. The first segment was 5.96 miles, and before I knew it, I was at the exchange. I passed my snap wrist band off to Jen for the second segment which was 5.83 miles.

She ran the entire segment, as I did. Her segment was a gradual uphill run. As each member of the team finished her segment, she had a story to tell in the van. Machelle had the next segment of 5.03 miles. It actually started to rain. Her segment was rolling uphill on Highway 75. She ran/walked her first segment. We did check on her once during her segment, and she said she was fine. So we headed to the next exchange point where the next three members of our team met us. They actually got to sleep a few more hours than we did. Lucky!

Tammy was the next member of the team to continue on a 4.43 mile segment. This segment was a gradual uphill on Highway 75. As Tammy started on her segment, we drove 30 minutes back to the hotel, showered, and took an hour plus nap. Then we returned to the course around 10:00 a.m. so our volunteer, Heidi, could get to exchange 11 to fulfill her job responsibilities. Amy took the next segment which was 5.83 miles. Her segment was a long steady uphill on the same highway. Carol took on the summit run. Her segment was 5.35 miles of nothing but a long, steady uphill, with curves and switchbacks. Her segment ended .15 mile past Galena Summit which was 8701 feet. It was regarded as one of the most difficult segments. The elevation gain during her ascent was 1, 331 feet.

Meanwhile, I sat on top of the mountain getting psyched for my next segment. The 7th leg was 6.02 miles and was a long, steady downhill with curves and switchbacks. The descent in elevation was

1411 feet. I could really feel my core muscles holding my body in the right position as I ran this segment. I finished my second leg very strong and felt good! I passed off to Jen who ran 5.09 miles on a steady downhill descent. She passed off to Machelle who ran the entire 4.64 miles on a moderate length leg, which was on a steady downhill. And here Machelle was worried about holding the team back with her 18 minute mile. She actually finished strong with a 14:29 mile average on the second leg. She wrote to me afterwards, "Did I do that? I can't believe I ran the whole leg." Machelle passed off to Tammy who did the longest segment at 6.13 miles on rolling downhills. Tammy then passed off to Amy who did 4.97 miles on a gradual downhill. While Amy was giving it her all, we all decided to go get coffee to recharge, and, yes, we did get one for Amy and Heidi. Amy passed off to Carol who walked the final 2.64 miles.

We also had a team photographer, Carrie, who was not able to get on a team. She took all our team photos, and walked with Carol on both her segments to experience what the race was like. Her participation was considered unofficial, but she was definitely part of our team! The entire team met Carol and Carrie about one mile from the finish line and we all walked in together.

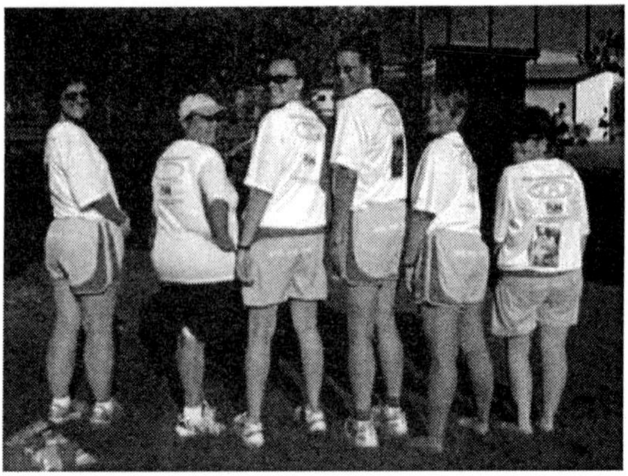

Machelle, Carol, Jen, Anita-Nell, Tammy, Amy.
Our butts have our team name "Going, Going....Gone"
Shorts donated by Dr. Oakley
Printing Donated by Athletic design

We did our finish-line pictures, and received our awards. The awards to this race are slightly different from other races. They give you a finisher memento, which is something given back from nature. We all received Heulandites Crystals that are produced by the Rat's Nest Mine in Custer County, Idaho, the only source for these crystals in North America. We each got a t-shirt and a bag of these crystals. Then the party began. We had some great music provided by Sonic Skillet, and a great gourmet meal of Clear Spring Trout, topped with cucumber dill yogurt, rosemary herb-roasted potatoes, Falls Brand Sausages, big 'ole bakery rolls, and some nice coleslaw. The meal was topped off with soft drinks, ale, and strawberry shortcake to boot!

The best part of a race like this is the true bonding experience you have with your teammates before, during, and after the race. All of us totally enjoyed the post race celebration. We sat in the park eating our gourmet meals and reflecting on our experiences. We all agreed to return the following year because of how much fun we had on the trip and race. A post-race story: On the way home, late at night, we passed one of those signs that say, "Next service 45 miles." I was not even paying attention, but my co-pilot did say 20 miles later, "You do realize you have no gas?" We ended up coasting downhill and praying for the next 25 miles. By the time we refilled at the next service, I only had two tenths of a gallon left in the tank. Wow, that was close!

Fit for Life 5K, 10K, and ½ Marathon

The following month on July 22nd my running club and weight loss support group runners all joined the 5K, 10K, and half marathon in the Fit for Life race. This is the big summer race in Idaho. My grand daughter Kelly, 11, came out to watch me in this race, and it made a big impact on her that her grandmother could complete a race of this size. Jen, Tammy, Machelle, and I all signed up for the half marathon. This would be the first half marathon for the other three. Jen and I decided to pair up since our paces were similar. For the first 6 miles we ran great together; averaging about 9:40 miles. Between miles 6-8 our time drastically changed to 14 minute miles. I was a little confused at the times, and asked Jen if she wanted to run ahead. I felt I was slowing us down.

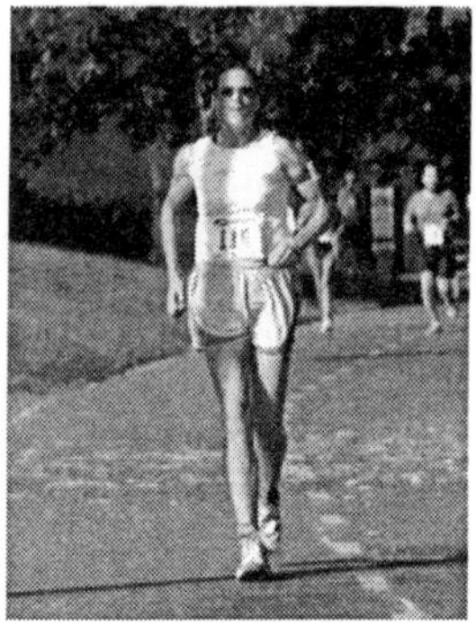

Fit for Life half Marathon.
(IdahoSportsPics)

As it turned out, the course was mislabeled and we ended up running over 3 miles between mile 6 and 8. I tried to catch up to Jen, but she kept running ahead. I could just keep her in my sights, and then when I rounded a corner, she would be gone. I arrived at the finish line, and found out that Jen had not yet crossed. I became a little panicked.

Our running coach, Steve, had brought his bike to the race, so he took off back-tracking the course. Before he could return, a clump of runners approached the finish line, and one of them was Jen. She was barely walking, and wiped out. As it turned out, she and the other runners had taken a wrong turn, and she ended up running a full 17.5 miles. She had never run over 9 miles. Two of us had to run out to Jen about a quarter of a mile from the finish line, and put her arms around our shoulders. We walked her to the finish line.

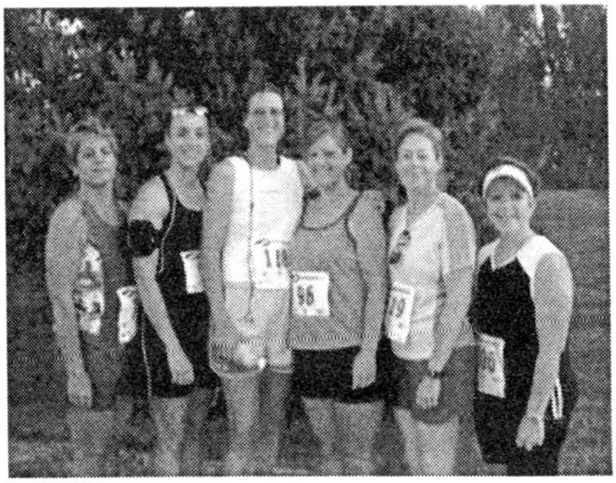

Tammy, Jen, Anita-Nell, Machelle, Colleen, and Amy.

Jen, who is the dietitian for our Gastric Bypass group, did not carry any spare water or nutrition on the course. So she not only became dehydrated, she had also depleted her electrolytes. On our way home she got sick. We were all really concerned and worried, and thought we would have to take her to the hospital. She was able to eat a banana and drink some water and the color began to return to her face. She seemed to recover after eating the banana and drinking the water. Now that she is okay, we still rib her about being the dietitian who did not take advice from fellow runners.

Disneyland Inaugural Race Weekend

In the second week of September I participated in the Inaugural Disneyland Pirates of the Caribbean 5K Fun Run and the Disneyland half marathon. We spent the first day at the parks, and the second day at the running expo, where we got our race packets. I went to bed early, and arrived at the staging area at 6:00 a.m. Saturday morning wearing my Goofy Pirates of the Caribbean hat to check in.

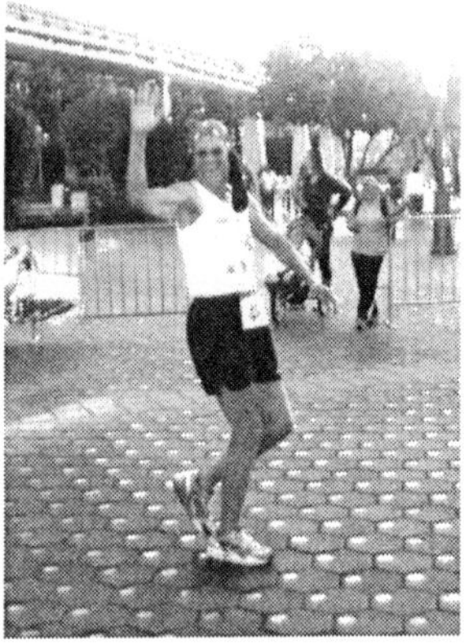

Disneyland Pirates of the Caribbean 5K Fun Run.

The race started at 7:00 a.m. We ran through Downtown Disney, through Disneyland, and then ended the race in Disney's California Adventure. This was a fun and exciting run and was a good preview to how the half marathon would be run through the different parks. This was the first time I ran in Southern California, so I wanted to get used to the weather and the air quality. At the finish line, Dale was waiting for me with a big hug. I received my medal, a skull and cross bone, and got my picture taken with the medal.

For the half marathon, I was joined by Malinda, her husband Hami, and her daughter-in-law, Savain. Hami was so impressed with Malinda and me at the last half marathon in Walt Disney World that it motivated him to join us for this race here in Disneyland. Lori from the Disney World race also joined us. No travel was required for her; she lived in Southern California.

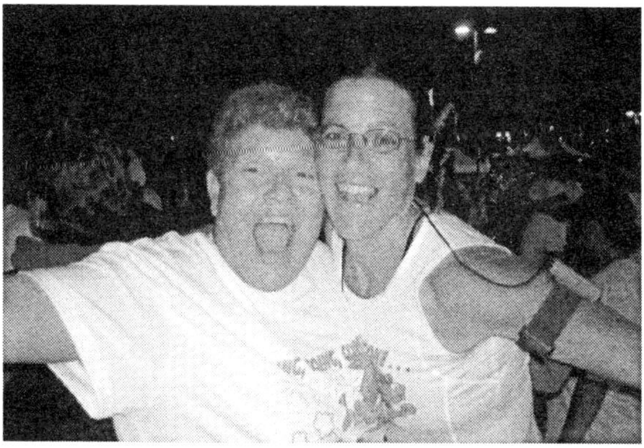

Malinda and I very excited prior to the half marathon.

We all met at 3:00 a.m. and hiked down to the staging area, where we met all our volunteer friends. The Disney pre-race announcer, got us all hyped up. It's amazing how many potable bathrooms are needed for 17,000 runners. At 5:00 a.m. we were asked to go to our corrals. This time I was in the right one. It was "A" corral, and Malinda, Hami, and Savain were further back in the pack. The starting line went under the monorail.

The monorail pulled up 30 minutes prior to the start. All the Disney characters hung out the windows and cheered everyone on as we were got ready for the race. Jeff Galloway, an Olympic Gold Medal runner, and a writer for *Runner's World*, was there to inspire the crowd. He is well-known for the Galloway run/walk method which has inspired the average person to run low mileage 3 days a week, and his program has an awesome 98 percent success rate. He actually ran the half marathon with us. Mickey and Minnie started the Inaugural Event and waved to us as we ran by.

I am such a slow starter. I totally took in the sights for the first 3 miles. We started on the streets of Anaheim, and circled around into California Adventure across the plaza to Disneyland and down Main Street. The course wound through Disneyland then exited Main Street and through downtown Disney to the streets of Anaheim where we passed by the frozen pond of the Anaheim Ducks, and continued to Anaheim Stadium. At the 3-mile marker, as I exited Disneyland, my pace was just over an 11 minute mile. So I took the opportunity to speed up on the stretch to the stadium. I knew I needed to average 10 minute to 10.5 minute miles if I was going to break my personal best.

The cool thing about running a Disney marathon is that every mile is marked with a balloon arch over the street, and each mile marker has a clock. So when I saw the balloons approaching, I would dramatically speed up my pace to help my time. Another exciting feature of the run was that you actually got to run through Anaheim Stadium. You entered from the outfield, and ran to home plate. They took a couple of pictures while we were in the stadium. After I exited the stadium, I passed by the 10 mile clock. I noticed that I was 3 minutes under my last year's time at Walt Disney World. I knew that I not only wanted to break my personal best but wanted to shatter it. Like a horse, when I was within 3 miles of the finish, I begin to boogie to the barn. I was in such a zone that when I ran through downtown Disney on my way to the finish line, I totally missed Dale. He was waving and yelling at me, and I didn't even hear him. I crossed the finish line with an all time personal best of 2 hours 17 minutes and 30 seconds. This meant I was 7 minutes and 32 seconds better than my previous best time! My last 3 miles were 9:42 miles.

At the start of the race Hami asked Malinda if she would wait for him and their daughter-in-law, and Malinda replied, "Heck no, I'm trying to break my personal best from last year," and away she went. Malinda finished the half marathon in 3 hours 8 minutes and 43 seconds with a 14:23 mile average, which was 12 minutes 34 seconds better than Walt Disney World where she averaged 15:22 miles. Lori, running her second half marathon, also did great. She finished in 2 hours 37 minutes 47 seconds which was a 12:02 average mile. She topped her personal best from Walt Disney World by 6 minutes and 51 seconds with an average mile of 12:33. Way to go, girls! Hami finished just under the allotted time of 3 hours and 30 minutes, and Savain finished after the allotted time. We went to the post race awards and had our pictures taken. This time we had our medals engraved with our official time, pace, and place in the race. This was something we did not know we could do when we ran the Walt Disney World half marathon.

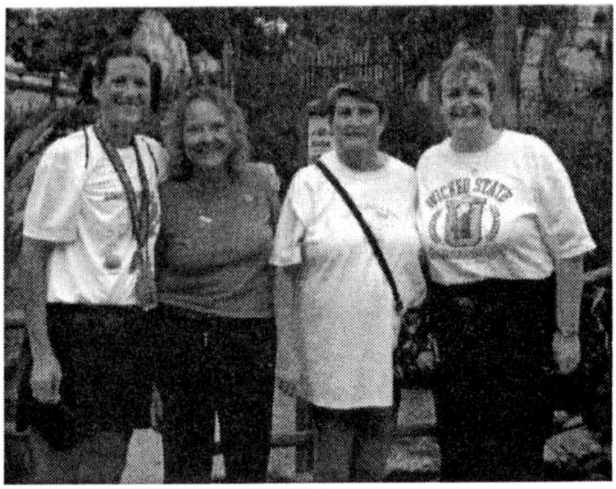

Wearing my medal proudly, and with Disney Pals and volunteers Dana Faith and Shari.

After running over mountains, running while ill, and on an extra long course in 100 degree heat, it was real refreshing to hit my personal best at the finish line. I was once again floating on air from this experience. I spent the rest of the day just enjoying myself, and doing Disneyland without a care in the world.

14th Annual St. Luke's 5K Women's Fitness Celebration

The following weekend I was in the St. Luke's 5K Women's Fitness Celebration for one reason and one reason only. I had challenged Machelle back during the Race for the Cure to run this race with me. I wanted her to run the entire 5K race. I told her I would help pace her throughout the race. Our goal would be to finish in 35 minutes, which is not a blistering speed. Machelle agreed to that challenge.

When I registered for this race, I also entered the Her Sports Giveaway from my favorite magazine. Would you believe it, I won the contest! I came home to an email that said, "Congratulations! You are the winner of the weekend getaway for two to St. Luke's 14th Annual Women's Fitness Celebration, in Boise, Idaho, September 21-23. Winner's package includes two VIP 5K entries, three-night hotel accommodations and an 'Experience Boise' package."

This package is just what I needed. It allowed me to have a few days of downtime that I so much needed (and didn't even know I needed). I was able to join the celebration with many friends and just enjoy being a woman. My husband and I were able to get some great downtime together on Saturday night and really enjoyed downtown Boise.

The morning of the race, Machelle, Linda, and I walked to the starting line with our husbands. When we got to the starting line we were met by the rest of our support group buddies, Tammy and her daughter-in-law, who was going to run/walk in the non-competitive purple wave, and Connie, who hooked up with Linda to walk in the competitive yellow wave. Machelle and I were going to run in the competitive red wave. Amy was going to run in the non-competitive purple wave. We couldn't find her before the race, but did find her later at the finish line.

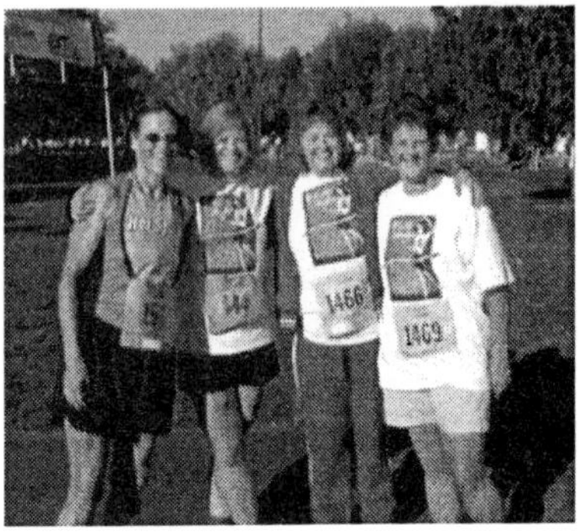

Anita-Nell, Machelle, Linda, and Connie.

As usual, they had great music at the start line. Machelle and I began to jump up and down and stretching before the starting gun. There were approximately 15 thousand runners entered in this race, and as I looked around the staging area I could see the different waves around me. Each wave starts to race at a different time. In front of me were all the handicapped athletes in wheelchairs. This group would start the race, then 5 minutes later the elite athletes would take off (about 20 elite runners), then 5 minutes later my red wave would leave, and so on. To the left of me was the purple wave, and to right was the yellow wave. These waves would leave after we did.

It is important to get your adrenaline pumped up prior to the start of a race. Machelle and I had succeeded in doing this, and we were both pumped up and ready to run. As the race began, I told her to take it slow and easy, and we would increase our speed as we went along.

Within half a mile of the start, Machelle said to me, "I am running faster than I have ever run before. I cannot do this." I kept constantly reassuring her that she could. We were on a small incline, so I would get her to focus on a small target ahead on the course. I would play a mental game with her. I would say, "Look up ahead, when we get to that light at the top of the incline, the course will flatten out, so grab your rope and pull yourself into that stop light." And then it was a tree, and then a stop sign. I wanted her to stop focusing on the speed of running, and just concentrate on portions of the course ahead. I wanted to teach her that breaking the run down into smaller portions or baby steps would make it easier to achieve, instead of constantly thinking about how much further we had to run. I knew we were up against the agreed goal time, so I constantly pushed Machelle so she would meet her goal.

Machelle did great; she was able to dig down deep to accomplish this goal! As we approached the finish line we could see the finish line clock. It had just rolled over to 35 minutes. I told Machelle that we needed to sprint if we were going to make it in time to meet the 35 minute goal. I did not want it to change to 36 minutes. So we sprinted and did make it in 35 minutes and some small change. Close enough, we hit our goal as far as I was concerned!

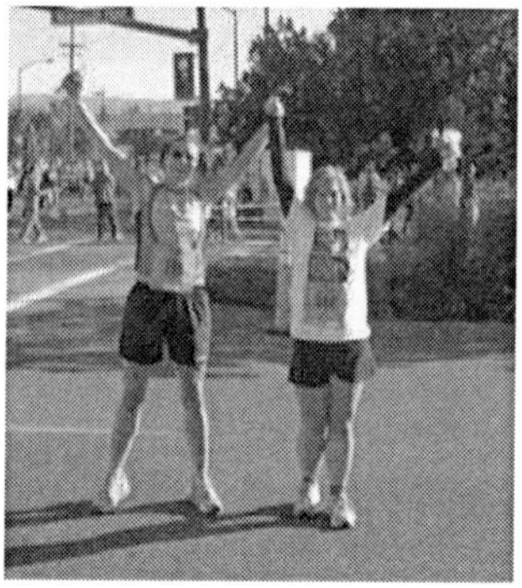

Machelle and I accomplishing our goal!

For Machelle it was exhilarating. She was able to celebrate that sense of accomplishment. I was very proud of her, and could not wait to run again with her. It was an unbelievable feeling to mentor, and pay it forward. I was so happy for Machelle and her experience.

After spending some time with me on the phone and hearing all about my weight loss journey, Loraine Oates, the head of the Celebration, decided to include me in an article to be written in our local Boise paper about three women. The article would be called, "Faces of Courage," and would include three profiles: the legend, the back-bone, and the inspiration. The segment of the article written about me was the inspiration. Members of the Montel Williams Show caught this story online. They asked me if I would come to New York and tell portions of my story for a show. I went to New York and did the Montel Williams Show, and hope the story I told there will inspire women everywhere to get healthy from the inside out!

Barber to Boise 10K

October 21st, just two weeks from my first full marathon, I entered this 10K to again mentor Machelle. My running coach Mike strongly advised me not to participate. However, Machelle felt she needed just one more running event prior to what would be her first half marathon as a runner. I promised my coach I was not going all out during the 6.2 mile event, and I was only there to help Machelle increase her distance running. So I agreed to pace Machelle one last time as a graduation to her first half marathon that she would do as a runner.

Justine, a member of our support group, also entered this event as a speed walker. We all decided to run together. Justine's fast walk is similar to Machelle's running speed. We took off together on the year's first real brisk autumn morning. As with the previous 5K, I spent a majority of the time reinforcing some of the same running techniques we used in the 5K. I tried to get Machelle to focus on short segments of the race by concentrating on things up ahead on the course like trees, signs, and street lights. I kept pointing to an object ahead and saying, "Come on Machelle just reel it in. Focus just on getting to that point."

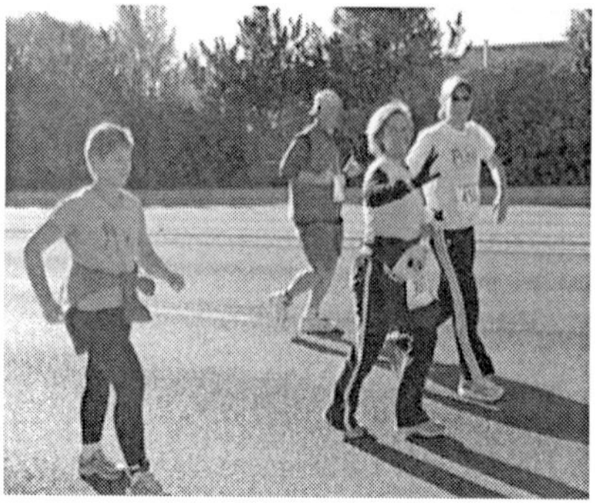

Barber to Boise Justine, Machelle, and Anita-Nell.

Around mile 4, we came across a woman running by herself. She saw the backs of our shirts and our weight loss pictures, and asked us what that was all about. Machelle explained our story as we ran, which made for an easy mile. I did not have to keep her focused at all. She talked and ran fine!

However, as we approached the end of the race, Machelle was ready to just walk in. Justine and I literally had to take her by the arms and pull her across the finish line.

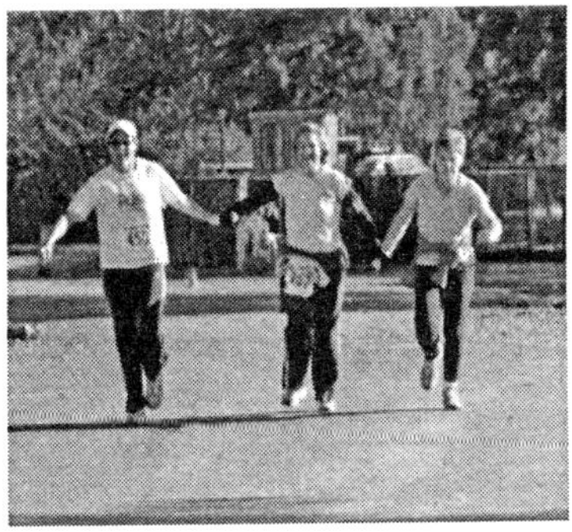

Pulling Machelle to the finish!
(IdahoSportsPics)

All in all, Machelle did real well. She was exited that she pushed herself to complete a 5K, and now a 10K. She was definitely ready to double the distance again, and run the half marathon in two short weeks. She was going to run her first half marathon with Linda, and I was going to run the full marathon. Reports came back to me that Machelle actually did real well in the half marathon, and was mentoring Linda with the same techniques that I had used with her. It is great to hear that after two races, she is already out there paying it forward. Way to go, Machelle!

As a side note, Steve, our head run coach of the BoiseRunWalk Club also ran this 10K, and he set a personal best for himself, and he came in first for his age group.

City of Trees Marathon

After I ran my first half marathon at Walt Disney World on my birthday in January 2006, I began to plan when I would run my first full marathon. I planned on returning to Walt Disney World on my following birthday and run the full marathon there. I then thought that on my birthday in 2008, I would return to Florida and run both the half and full marathon, all in one weekend. However, as my training progressed, after I joined the running club, and entered quite a few challenging races, I decided to step up these dates. Down deep inside I wanted to share the first-time experience of running a full marathon with my parents. This was becoming very important to me as I progressed in the running world. I knew I would not get my parents to join me in January all the way in Florida, especially since my mother's career is preparing income taxes, and her season begins January 1st. So I decided to change my first marathon to a local Idaho race called the City of Trees Marathon, which is run in the First week in November. I thought it would be much easier to bring my parents to Idaho than have them travel clear across the country.

When I first signed up for this race, I entered it as a half marathon, but once I saw how well my training was going, I decided to make this my big landmark race for my parents to witness. As it turned out, I flew to New York to be taped on the Montel Williams Show just 10 days before this race, and the day my parents arrived in Idaho for the race was the air date for the Montel Show. Within two hours after my parents arrived, we joined members of my support group and my running club to watch the show be aired for the first time at my house. It was a "Montel Party!" My parents got to meet a lot of my friends and running partners. It was awesome that my parents were able to meet people from my "NEW" life.

On Saturday I spent the day with my Mom. It was her birthday. We went to breakfast at my favorite restaurant, "Goldie's," and then we attended the "City of Trees" Expo, where I picked up my marathon running packet. I was able to have my favorite sweet potato hash browns and cheese and garlic omelet. My Mom got to see some of my friends from Thursday's party and a ton of other friends. We did a little shopping, and then went on a bus ride which drove the entire marathon course. We both took notes. For me it really helped in my mental preparation. I was able to pick out key landmarks for my run with performance goals around the course. I calculated places on the course where I would take my electrolyte replacements. My mom picked out different spots where she could watch the race. She did not realize how far 26.2 miles was when zigzagging in and out of the city streets. So it was absolutely fantastic they offered this bus service.

I religiously studied my notes that night and the morning of the race. It was great to add this step into my pre-race preparation. Saturday was such a gorgeous sunny day. I prayed for the same on Sunday, but a cold front rolled in overnight, and it began to rain by early morning. I recall hearing it tap on our skylights when I woke up. The forecast for the day was continuous rain. When I arrived at the staging area, it was cold and wet. I did not have rain gear for the run, so I poked three holes in a garbage bag, and wore it as my makeshift rain jacket. A lot of runners were in the same boat as I, and did the same thing. My mom was worried because of the rain, but I assured her I had run in the rain before, but I did pray that it did not rain for the whole day.

Instead of gathering at the starting line, we stayed under cover for most of the morning waiting for the race to start. I finally lined up with the BoiseRunWalk Club red runners; we were all going to pace together. As we got going at the start, we all stayed pretty bunched up, but by mile 7, four of us were way out in front of the other runners in the club. Jay, one of the runners in our club, said we should wait for the rest of the pack. He said, "We should all cross the finish line together. Who cares if we don't finish in 5 hours?" I knew in my head that statement would not hold up. Even if we waited for the rest of the pack, I believed that when we all got to the 13 mile point, everyone was going to take off on their own pace anyway. But I fell for Jay's argument, so we decided to wait. We first slowed down, then stopped, and slowly started running back on the course. We finally found the rest of the club. I have to tell you, waiting was a mistake. As we waited our muscles cooled down, so by the time the rest of the runners caught up, we had a hard time getting going again. Two of the runners we waited for actually passed right on by and never looked back. The muscles in my legs did not warm back up until mile 15 and I did not even get back into my groove until mile 20.

Major lesson learned: Do not stop for an extended period of time during a race. If you are running as a mentor, it is okay to take it easy, but if you are doing the race for yourself, your full concentration needs to be on your race and not on someone else's location during the race. One of the guys in our club almost fell off a curb, because the muscles in his leg cramped up too tight. I tried to help, but he decided to drop out. He could not get stretched out enough to get rid of the cramp, so I had to leave him behind. He never finished the marathon.

My parents and Dale drove around to different parts of the course. They were all great support on this cold and rainy day. Every time I was having a bad time, Dale was there with the van to give me fresh gloves, a sports drink for electrolytes, or a banana. My dad even came on the course and ran a short distance with me to pump me up. I would be lying if I said that it was just rain drops in my eyes. I couldn't help but cry. The volunteers on the course also did a great job keeping us going with their cheers and occasional hugs.

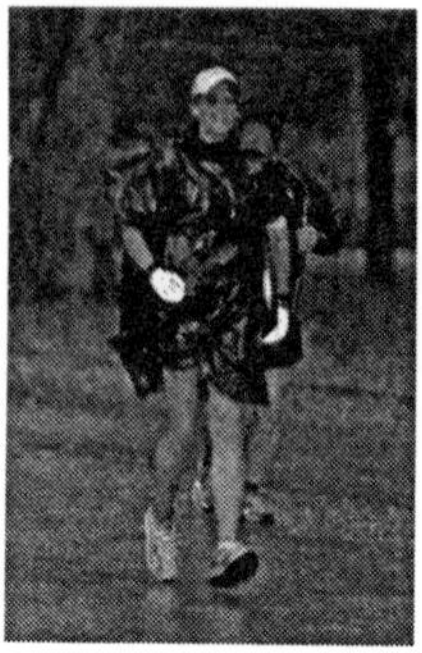 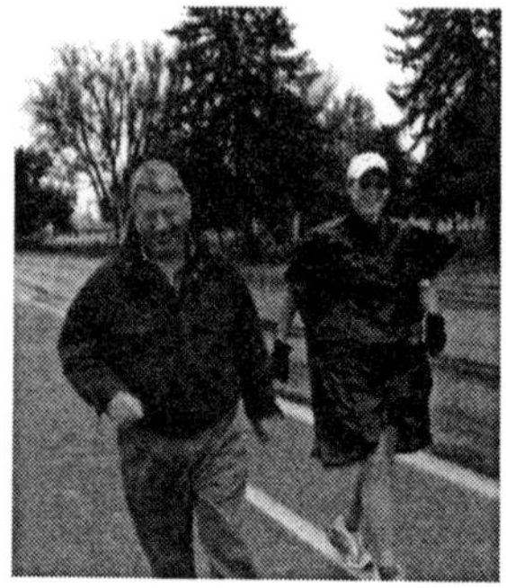

Running with my garbage bag since it rained all day.
My dad running with me for support.
(Left picture – IdahoSportsPics)

My original trainer and friend Jolene from the "Y" also came to the race. I had no idea she was there. I did invite her to come, but I didn't know if she made it or not. She camped out at the finish line, and was waiting for me to come in and cross the line.

As I got within the final 2 miles, I stripped my garbage bag off, picked up the pace, and headed to the "barn." When the finish line was within sight, I gave it my all and started to sprint. As I approached the finish line I could see my support group. I could see Dale, Mom, Dad, and then Machelle, and Linda, who had already finished their half marathon, Colleen, Donna, my coach Steve, my trainer Jolene, and others all there just sitting out in the rain waiting for me to finish. I also saw Kim and Carolyn from Pulse Fitness in Meridian who has supported me with encouragement since the day I met them. (They also sponsored our Sawtooth Relay team). I could not believe how loved I felt at that very moment. I was in awe! It was so awesome....what a reward!!! At the finish line, I was able to visit with everyone, and get my picture taken with all my supporters.

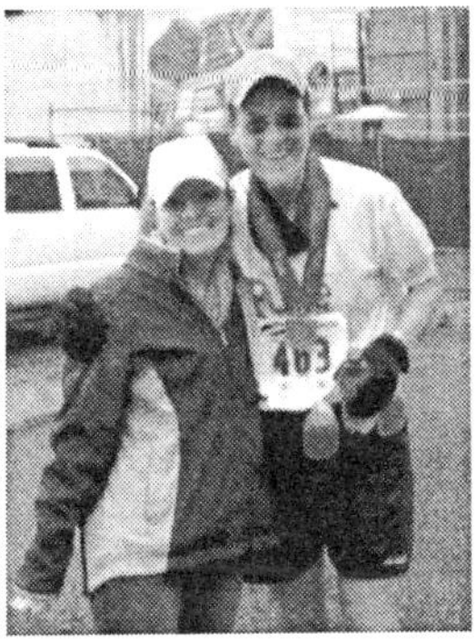

Jolene (my first personal fitness trainer) met me at the finish line. She was the spark to my fitness, and laid the foundation to my new life of running, and for that I am forever grateful. Thank You!

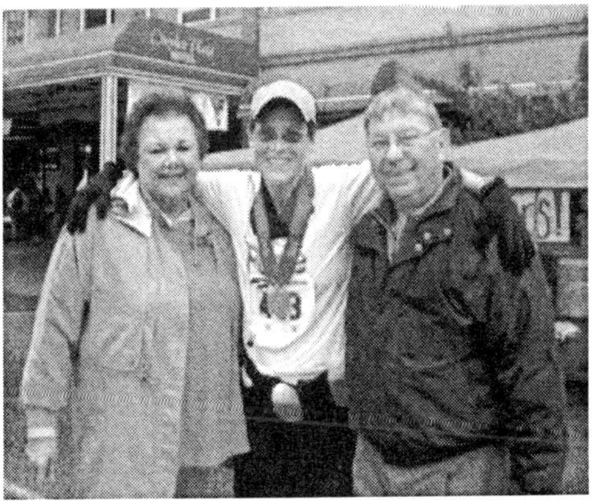

My mom and dad witnessed my first full marathon, and they met me at the finish line – Thank You!

My coach Steve presented me with a coach's hat for the BoiseRunWalk Club. This meant that I would now mentor and help coach the new marathoners starting this winter. Jolene was so proud of my effort, and could not believe how strong I finished. So in the rain, soaking wet, after stopping for others, and trying to help others continue, I was able to run the 26.2 miles in 5 hours and 27 minutes.

This was my last big race of the year. In my first 11 months of running, I had completed 11 events, including two half marathons and one full marathon. I will start 2007 at Walt Disney World in Florida with the first event of the year on the weekend of my birthday. It is called the "Goofy's Challenge," and includes the half marathon on Saturday and the full marathon on the following day. I am so psyched to do it.

I plan on running many of the same events in 2007; however, at the end of the year; I would like to run either the New York City marathon in November or the Chicago marathon in October. I haven't determined which one yet. I have already planned to do five different Rock 'N Roll Marathons in 2008. I plan on running Phoenix in January, Nashville in April, San Diego in June, Philadelphia and Virginia Beach in September, and San Jose in October. In 2009 my goal is to run the entire Sawtooth relay solo for all 62 miles as an Ultra Marathon.

I am so glad for all the coaching and help I have received over the last year. I totally appreciate it. I hope to see all of you soon on some of these courses.

Chapter 18

Kettlebells - It's a Goofy Thing

A kettlebell is an ancient cast-iron weight used by Russian Olympic Athletes, and later by Russian Special Forces. It was an intricate part of their weight training programs. It looks like a cannon ball with an attached handle. The typical weight of a kettlebell is 16 kg which is 36 pounds. The weight lifters in Russia typically used 16, 24, or 32 kg kettlebells in their weight lifting programs.

Lately, kettlebells are being used in fitness workouts in the United States. The workouts are designed to help you work all your muscles and help to strengthen and develop your core muscles. However, the kettlebell weights in these fitness programs are much lighter than their Russian predecessors. They normally are 4, 8, 12, and 16 kg, or 9, 18, 27, and 36 pounds.

Kettlebells have recently been written up in *Fitness Magazine* and *Tennis Magazine* as an alternative workout program. They benefit runners, tennis players, and any athlete who wants a workout to help strengthen their core muscles. They also benefit the everyday person because they work the muscles you use every day.

I was first introduced to kettlebells in one of my weekly BoiseRunWalk Club seminars. Kim, the owner of PowerHouse Pilates in Boise, presented the seminar. The demonstration was just an introduction to the kettlebells workout, which she promised would benefit your functional muscles. She explained that when you lift or work out at the gym, you usually work out just your large muscle groups, but not the functional muscles that you use on a daily basis. The benefit of a kettlebell workout is that it forces the functional muscles to be used. We were offered a free demonstration of the kettlebells after our run that day. I tried them out after we returned from our run. As with everything, I was a bit skeptical, and was not too sure how these weights were actually going to help me. I had already reached my goal weight, and I was running. This seemed to be overkill, so I procrastinated on any further investigation for a while.

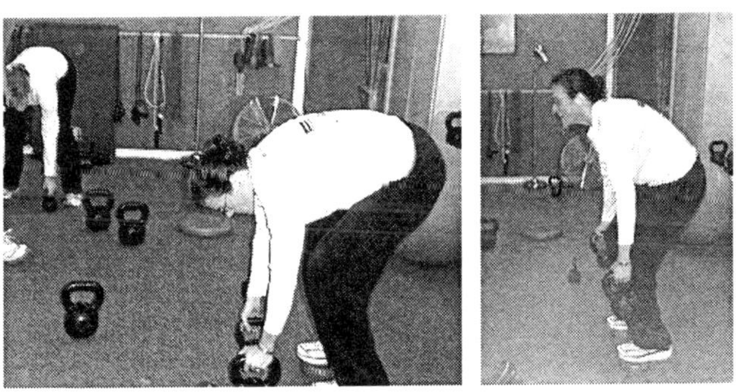

Working out with kettlebells.
Powerhouse Pilates, Boise Idaho

I began to ask other runners over the summer how the kettlebell workouts were helping them with their running. All of them said it was making their runs easier on their muscles. So in September before my

Inaugural Disneyland Race, I decided to sign up for some classes. I believe I was able to get four kettlebell classes in prior to the Disneyland half marathon. I remember feeling great during the race, and setting a personal best record. I was convinced that my kettlebell workouts were what helped me, so I continued to take the classes at PowerHouse Pilates Studio after I returned from Disneyland.

When I first began kettlebell workouts, I was working out three days a week at the YMCA with weights. So I traded one of my YMCA workout days to do kettlebells once a week. I started to notice that not only was my running improving with each race, but my soreness or tiredness after each race became less and less over time. I totally attribute this to the kettlebell training. I stopped kettlebells one week prior to my first marathon, and I noticed the difference. I was not as sore after that race.

As time went on, I swapped two of my workout days at the YMCA for kettlebells. So I now work out twice a week with the kettlebells and once a week with weights at the "Y." I have total belief and confidence in the kettlebell fitness program. I recently ran my first half and full marathon on the same weekend, without any negative side effects or soreness. I know I could not have done this without the kettlebell training.

Goofy's Challenge

This race weekend was my first running goal of 2007. It was the running of a half marathon on Saturday, the day before my birthday, and then running the full marathon on my birthday, on Sunday. Yep, you run both in the same weekend in Florida's Walt Disney World. Disney calls that the Goofy's Challenge when you do both the half and the full marathon in the same weekend.

I ran with my friends Donna and Colleen from BoiseRunWalk Club. Donna did the Goofy Challenge, and Colleen ran the half Marathon. We had all trained together for these races for the past two months. I was torn wondering if I should run the half and full marathons for my personal best time, or if I should run just an average pace. I finally decided that any time I do a race with the name Disney in it; I'm just going to soak up the moment and have fun. Running alongside and around Disney characters is truly meant to be fun. So that is what I did.

The day of the half marathon we all started from different corrals. My only race goal was to maintain 12 minute miles and to have fun. We didn't see each other through the entire half marathon, but we all had a fun time.

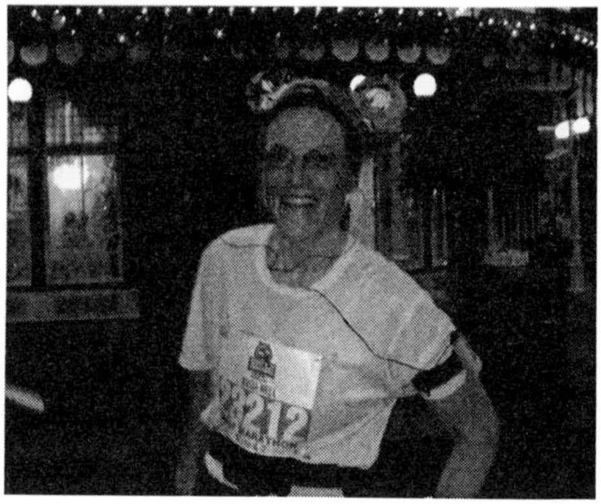

Running down Main Street during the half marathon.

On the next day, Donna and I decided to run the marathon together as long as we could keep the same pace. Her husband is named Chip, and of course mine is Dale. So we did stop to get our picture taken together with the Disney characters Chip and Dale.

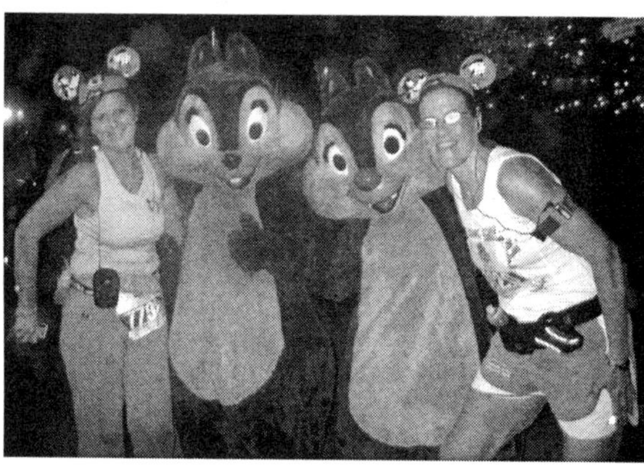

With Chip and Dale.

Everything was great from the starting line until we left Epcot. Between Epcot and the Magic Kingdom I lost sight of Donna for a little bit, but we met back up to run through the Magic Kingdom together. We were able to run together through the front 13.1 miles. Donna had to stop for a pit stop, and we weren't able to meet up again for the rest of the race. I got a lot of pictures taken with Disney Characters and animals (including a turtle, an alligator, a hawk, and a macaw) as I ran through the Animal Kingdom.

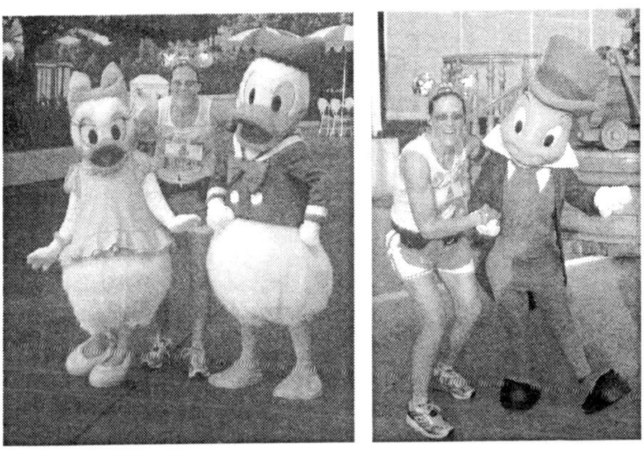

Me with Daisy Duck, Donald Duck, and Jiminy Cricket.

It was a hot day with high humidity, and two water stations in a row ran out of water, so I walked a portion of the course until the next water station so I could get re-hydrated.

We ran through the Boardwalk and back to Epcot at the end where we ran around the world and all the countries, and then under the big ball at the finish line. In the last 3 tenths of a mile I kicked into my strong finish mode. I must have passed 50 people as I weaved in and out to the finish line. I felt real good, and I was able to cool down real quickly.

I went to the post race event and received my medals. With the Goofy Challenge you receive three medals: one for the half marathon, one for the full marathon, and a Goofy Medal for completing both marathons in the same weekend.

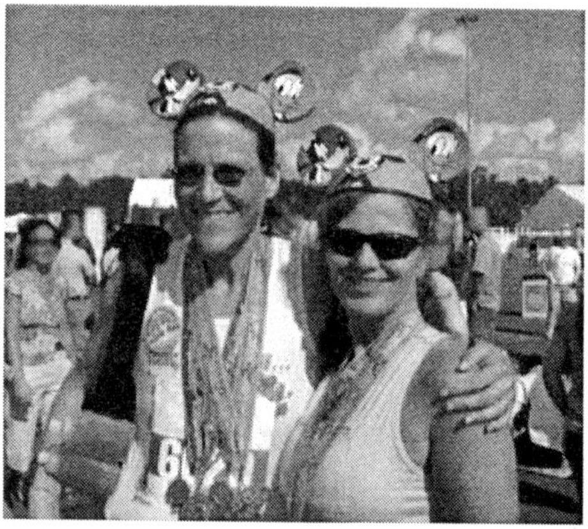

Donna and I after the Goofy Challenge with our medals.

I felt great after the race. We went out that night and I had tons of energy the next day when I flew home. I was running up and down the stairs at the airport because I felt so great. I was not sore at all!

I had actually finished this book prior to the Goofy's Challenge, but felt compelled to add my experiences from it to the book along with the information on my kettlebells training. I truly believe that my lack of sore muscles in this last race was solely because of my kettlebell training.

Whether you choose to run or not, I still think you should look into a kettlebell class in your area. It is well worth your time and energy. You can also get more information about kettlebells with an online search or going to http://www.pwrhousepilates.com.

Chapter 19

Inspiration and Pay it Forward

Out of all the chapters in this book, this one is the most important, and is closest to my heart. Whether it is weight loss, weight loss surgery, or even running a marathon, a person needs to have inspiration and support from others to succeed.

Inspiration is the reason we do what we do. We become inspired from others before us, so we too have hope that we can do the same.

My first inspiration, when I took control of my life and started to lose my initial 135 pounds, was Bill Phillips, and his book, *Body for Life*. After seeing the Montel and Oprah shows on television, and reading Bill's book, I began the first steps in becoming healthy from the inside out. I was truly inspired. The next big inspiration I had was at my first support group meeting, prior to my surgery, when I overheard those two ladies talking about how easy it was for them to climb stairs. Also, Jolene, my first fitness trainer, was a huge inspiration to me. And there were countless others along my weight loss journey too numerous to mention here, but who have continued to inspire me.

I cannot count how many times there was someone there to take me to the next place or to the next level. It was not always the same person; it was different people for my different needs. From some people I just needed their inspiration for a moment, and others have touched my life, and I will be friends with them forever.

Several years ago I saw a movie titled *Pay It Forward* with Kevin Spacey and Helen Hunt. (The movie was based on *Pay It Forward*, a novel by Catherine Ryan Hyde.) I love this concept and I have tried to apply this principle to my life. Since I was able to go through the surgery and successfully lose 230 pounds from the Gastric Bypass, I have always felt an obligation, to pay it forward to others who want to lose a massive amount of weight. I want to be able to pass on to them what I learned. I want to be their inspiration, and I want to help them through their weight loss journey. Whether it is someone needing help adjusting to their new life and way of eating, or going on a walk, or helping them out at the gym, I feel a responsibility to help them. Even if I'm tired and just want to go home, I feel it is more important to help, and I always feel better after I do.

I get emails all the time thanking me for some act I performed in helping someone, and they always ask if there is anything they can do for me. I always reply to their emails and say, "Just pay it forward." Someday, someone is going to need your help, or might be having a hard time, and so I only ask that you help them out and "pay it forward."

As you may have read in the previous running chapters, I have mentored several women from my support group when they've been learning to run. Now they have begun to mentor others. It is all about being able to live a healthy life, and passing on what we have learned to others. It is a very simple concept, and it is my hope and dream that all who have been successful with the weight loss surgery will help the next generation and beyond as they begin their weight loss journey.

I thought I would end this chapter and book with some inspirational writings I have received from others.

Below is an email I received from my Aunt Judy after a retreat we attended together four months before my surgery. It touched me and was a true inspiration to continue with my weight loss journey.

Anita-Nell,

I am writing this email in love; please take it in that concept. I just listened to the news and there was a report about the problems in our country, and number one was the obesity issue. I saw this week-end the Anita-Nell I did not know, a person so loving and so generous with her time, it blew me away. You have the most outreaching heart, I was in awe!! You are such a loving person. God has given you the ability to be so special in other's lives and it sure showed this week-end. I love you, and I want you to be around to continue to give your love to others. I want Karlee to have the grandmother of all grandmothers for the majority of her life. You will be there for her and help her in ways you don't even know right now. Please continue to follow your diet program, and become healthy. Your weight has never been a problem with me and my feelings for you. I would love you no matter what, but I want to tell you that you have sooooooo much to offer and you need to stay healthy to do it. Use any of us for support, we are here.

I had such a great time with you and Johnnie this week-end. I think I could sit and talk to you for hours. You are a great listener; you stay silent, and look into the person's eyes. That is the signal of "I care what you are saying." Anita-Nell, you are a gift from God. I see Grandpa Brown (Harry) in you; you have the genuine gift of God's love in your heart.

I told Gary I want to come over to visit you guys. He agreed. You and Johnnie are such assets to our family and always make our family gatherings more fun.

So keep up your good work on losing weight and working out. I know it is hard, so hard, but I want you to do it for yourself, for me and your granddaughters, for Dale, and for yourself.

Email me any time if there is anything I can do or say. This past week-end was a gift to me; I got to see you and Johnnie as true Christians with so much to offer.

Love in Christ,
Aunt Judy

Below is an email I received from Amy, who did the Minnie Marathon with me in May of 2006. She was the first support group member to run with me at a running event. This email was prior to the event. Amy ended up running both the 5K and 15K. And I am happy to report she is currently losing weight.

Hi, Anita-Nell,

I did a full five days last week. On Saturday, I did the whole 5K and it wasn't actually that difficult. I'm slow, but steady. I'm surprised that I could even do it. I did it in 40 minutes.

Tonight (Tuesday), I didn't even want to run...but got on the treadmill anyhow. I had a FANTASTIC run. I stopped at 35 minutes, but I could have kept going easily.

I have no more shin splints...so far. I've lost no weight yet...but the running is definitely getting easier. I have been considering running the 15K at WDW. Because it's an inaugural event...and the only way you get the Minnie Mouse medal is by doing the 15K...I think I'll try to go for it. I already signed up and paid for the 5K.

I can't thank you enough for giving me this opportunity. Not only is it awesome to hit DW and the new Expedition Everest ride and all...but I'm REALLY stoked about exercising! I needed this kick in the butt. I guess I need to look for another running goal for this summer so I don't lose it after the Minnie Marathon. Who knows, maybe you'll see me running the half marathon at DW in January... ha-ha :)

Later,
Amy

Next is an email I received from Colleen who is also from my support group. She had just tried out the BoiseRunWalk Club, and she very exited. She has since joined, and she also got her friend Jill to join too! So she is now paying it forward. Way to go!

Hey, Anita-Nell-

I just wanted to take a moment to thank you. Surprisingly, I had a really good time on Saturday. I was amazed that I didn't get a headache later that day like I normally do and that I wasn't sorer on Sunday, but Hey! I'm good with that. That is usually one of my biggest struggles when I start working out again - the headaches. I really like the pace we kept at the start of the run and feel very happy after completing 8 miles. I went to a barbeque later in the day with my co-workers and Jill, who I run with during the week, was amazed that I completed 8 miles and was still walking - and smiling! She is planning to join us next Saturday to check it out.

You are such a great inspiration. I really appreciate all your support and encouragement. You really are a special person. I'm lucky to know you.

Let me know if there is a plan for Saturday. I would love it if we could do something like we did last Saturday. That worked out nicely, provided Machelle and Linda don't mind the company.

Anyway, thanks again! I hope you know what a gift your encouragement has been to me.

Have a great week! Colleen

Below is an email my running coach Steve received on my behalf from Jose, who presented me with an award for “Outstanding Performance Road Racing 2005/2006.” I was not able to receive this award personally, so my friend Machelle received it on my behalf.

Dear Steve,

Thank you very much for allowing me to borrow your sound system. It was really a popular item in the race.

I also wanted to thank you for sharing the story of

one of your runners, Anita-Nell Swanson. Her story was very inspirational and touching to all who attended the race. I am sure that many (including me) will think of her when finding some rough times and stones on the road.

Touching and inspiring people, I believe, is the most important element in any race/event. It is great when someone like Anita-Nell can touch someone and inspire a group of people so they can reach their full potential as athletes and human beings. After beginning just a little over a year ago to become fit, this past Saturday she shared a spot with some of the finest athletes in our State. Her friend Machelle was there to claim her award.

Tentatively, the RWTA 2007 will take place on September 15th, 2007, and the theme will be the Olympic Games. I will try to prepare something for all participants so they can start celebrating such a great event.

Thank you again, Steve,

Jose Fuentes
NYK Line (NA), Inc.

The following email I received from Linda who I helped mentor on how to run/walk. I also got her started in her competitive walking. She ended up doing a half marathon at the Fit for Life race.

Anita-Nell,

Great job on the race! I think you're getting me hooked! That was fun competing with the clock and I'm totally stoked on entering another one as long as it's timed! It helps to know that I walked it faster than I thought I did. I thought I did 15.62 minute miles and it was 14.93. I think I might have been able to walk a little faster if I'd tried harder; you can bet next time I will. I actually wanted to jog if you can believe that. But I stuck to the rules and only walked. ***Can you believe what YOU started!*** *It was fun to see the results. Connie and I were in the top third (almost the top 25) and I was worried that we'd be near the last.*

You were right about the adrenaline kicking in when others are out there competing too. I know that I normally walk about 17.5 to 18 minute miles when I'm walking by myself or with Machelle. That's why I thought I'd be near the last. There might actually be two teams competing in the Sawtooth Relay Race since you're getting so many people started with racing.

We all need to get together sometime.

Anyhoo, I'd better get back to work.

Linda

Below are a few excerpts from Machelle's profile on Obesityhelp.com

5/21/06 - *Lots has happened in the past 11 days. I'm still "training" for the Sawtooth Relay. I did my first 5K (3.1 miles). It was in the Susan G. Komen Race for the Cure on Saturday, May 13. Two of my support group buddies (Anita-Nell and Linda) joined me and we walked/jogged it in 45 minutes. It was a huge self-confidence builder. Without Anita-Nell, Linda and I would have just walked it; but Anita-Nell is an amazing role model and motivator. Since she has gone from 527 pounds to 165 pounds, I can't seem to make any excuses for not doing what she asks of me. She is very positive and has a huge heart.*

Linda is so supportive of me and the three of us together got into the spirit of the race and encouraged each other throughout it. I'm so blessed to have these two as my friends. Anyway, Anita-Nell has been encouraging me to begin running, so during the race, she had the chance to watch me try my hand at jogging. She told me that I have good form and am holding my body right. That was so important for me to hear. Last Thursday, I got up the confidence to try Anita-Nell's 3-2-1 walk/jog training method. In this method, you walk for 3 minutes, jog for 2, walk for 1, jog for 3, walk for 2, jog for 1,etc. I didn't think I could run for 2 minutes, let alone 3, but I did it. The hardest part was jogging 2 minutes, walking 1 minute and then jogging 3 with such a short break in between. I'm sure a year from now, I'll think "what a wimp I was" because I thought this was hard. Anyway, I walked a total of 4 miles, but did the 3-2-1 thing for 2-1/2 of those miles. My knee was really hurting the next day though. I may have tried to go too far too soon.

9/23/06 *- Today was another milestone day for me. Four months ago (in May), Anita-Nell challenged me to run the St. Luke's Women's 5K on this date. I'm not sure why she did that because I barely knew her at the time. I have been so blessed by her friendship and support. At the time that she gave me the challenge, I had not even began to run and I sincerely doubted I could do this. Well, even though I've run/walked the Race for the Cure (5K), Sawtooth Relay (10 miles in 2 legs), and Fit for Life (13.2 miles), this race was a challenge to me. I had run more than 3 miles in the Sawtooth Relay, but I did that without any real concept of the distance I was running and I could allow myself to walk any time I wanted to. This race, I HAD to run within 35 minutes and with my exercise routine greatly compromised this summer, I felt challenged to a different level. Could I really run less than a 12-minute mile? I had to believe I could.*

11/05/06 *- You know how someone says something and it hits your heart and really means something personally to you? Well, two things Anita-Nell said on the Montel show have stuck with me all week. In her opening segment, Anita-Nell said "I feel like my body has been healed from the inside out because I put good food in it, and I've exercised, and I've* *created a lot of really good habits." In the past few weeks, I have struggled with cravings for Halloween candy and felt like it would be so easy to slide back into old habits now that I am eating "normally." Each day, I picture Anita-Nell on TV saying "I've created a lot of really good habits," and I know that in the past 18 months, I too have developed healthy habits. The second thing she said that struck home was, "I didn't want to be that person any more." I also don't ever want to "be the person I was before" and to not go there, I know that I can't revert back to the bad eating habits that consumed my past life and made me depressed, sick, and tired. Indulging in candy over Halloween reminded me just how tired and yucky I used to feel eating like that. So, now, when those ugly head hunger issues arise and the devil tempts me, I think about a segment in Bill Phillips' book about eating being a natural instinct that people have to battle. He says men by nature are hunters and gatherers of food and I say to myself, "I can fight this, because over the past 18 months, I too have developed healthy habits that will see me through the rest of my life."*

Today was my half-marathon run in the City of Trees Marathon. I was indifferent about signing up for it more than a month ago, but last night I was so excited about the race that I could hardly get to sleep. I woke up excited and feeling good. My daughter marched in the Veterans Day Parade for JROTC yesterday and the streets were wet, but the weather was nice and clear. With the sun drying out the streets and only a 30 percent chance of rain, I expected a beautiful day for my race. I was really bummed to wake up and see it raining outside. We were told at the start of the race that it was the race's 5th year and it was the 5th year of bad weather. (Next year they are moving the race to October.) It poured rain throughout the whole race. I was completely soaked from head to toe, clear through to my underclothes - and I was even wearing a poncho. My hair was drenched and I could wring water from it. I was okay though because it wasn't windy and cold while I was running. I did get very cold though after the race standing in my wet clothes waiting for Anita-Nell to finish her marathon. It was great to be a part of this important day for her - her first marathon and her parents were here to watch her run the first time. I started the race with my walking/training buddy, Linda. We stayed together until about mile 5 and then we both finished the race on our own. I am so proud of Linda. This was her first half marathon and, although it was hard on her, she persevered and made it through. She has more gumption than most women I know. At about mile 6-1/2, I walked with a marathoner who wasn't doing too well. He needed some food and I had extra with me, so I gave him a protein bar. I later told the paramedics to watch for him as he was behind me. He passed me about 3 miles from the end of the race - the protein bar must have really helped him. It made me feel good that the Lord used me to help someone finish his first marathon. I wish I could have seen him at the finish line, but he finished before I ever got there. My race time could have been better, but I'm okay with it. I finished in 3 hours, 16 minutes (14.98 minute miles) - less than my first half marathon three months ago. I had more energy at the end of the race and wasn't hurting and "wiped out" afterwards. That was a great feeling! Colleen ran the half marathon as well and it was nice to spend time with her today. Anita-Nell had quite a welcoming party at the end of the race. That was nice!

Thanks for taking the time to read my story. It has been a long and winding journey for me. However, I hope my story and this book have inspired you, or someone you know, to lose weight and become healthy too from the inside out. Please "pay it forward" and help others along the way; enjoy and celebrate life as I am.

- Anita-Nell -

Appendix

Useful Website Links:

ObesityHelp.com
http://www.obesityhelp.com

My Surgeon:
W. Christian Oakley, M.D.
http://www.Thinidaho.com

U.S. Department of Health and Human Services
http://www.hhs.gov/

NIDDK - The National Institute of Diabetes and Digestive and Kidney Diseases
http://www2.niddk.nih.gov/

BMI Calculator
http://www.nhlbisupport.com/bmi/

The American Society for Bariatric Surgery (ASBS)
http://asbs.org/

The Society of American Gastrointestinal and Endoscopic Surgeons
http://www.sages.org/

Find a YMCA near you:
http://www.ymca.net/

Kettlebells
http://www.pwrhousepilates.com
http://en.wikipedia.org/wiki/kettlebell

Local Supporters:

The Pulse Running and Fitness Shop
http://www.racingpulse.com

Athletes Foot Boise
http://www.athletesfootboise.com

Therapeutic Associates
http://www.therapeuticassociates.com/Locations/clinic.aspx?id=62

BoiseRunWalk Club
http://www.Boiserunwalk.com

St Luke's Fitness Challenge
http://www.celebrateall.org

Interest:

Pay It Forward
This site tells about the book which inspired the movie.
Cathrine Ryan Hyde. Author of "Pay it forward"
http://www.payitforwardmovement.org/

Montel Williams Show: I had my first guest appearance on November 2, 2006.
http://www.montelshow.com/

Oprah Winfrey Show: If you were inspired because of my book, please let Oprah know.
http://www2.oprah.com/

Recommended Reading:

Title: *Body for Life*
Author: Bill Phillips / M. D'Orso
Publisher: Harper Collins/Markets

Title: *Weight Loss Surgery: Finding the Thin Person Hiding Inside*
Author: Barbara Thompson
Publisher: Word Association

Magazines:

Her Sports + Fitness Magazine
http://hersports.com/

Obesity Help Magazine
http://obesityhelp.com/magazine/

Runner's World Magazine
http://www.runnersworld.com/

Sponsorships:

Athletic Design
458 N Fulton
Fresno, CA 93701
1-559-485-4673

Thanks To Malinda and Hami at Athletic Design for putting our team name on our shorts.

Thanks to Kim and Carolyn at pulse fitness and running shop for supplying our team shirts.

Thanks to Dr Oakley for supplying our team shorts.

Disney Marathons

http://disneyworldsports.disney.go.com

Click - Headline Events
Click - Walt Disney World Marathon Weekend, or Disneyland Half Marathon Weekend

Referenced Material

Chapter 10
Dr. Oakley, "Request and Informed Consent Form" (2004) 1-3, "Binding Obesity Contract" (2004) 1-2, "Obesity Surgery Patient Exam" (2004) 1-1.

Leah H Davidson, "Giving Me Life", poem, (2004) 1-1

Chapter 11
http://www.obesityhelp.com, author unknown, Term of Morbid Obesity, (2006)
Dr. Oakley, "Nutritional Guidelines After Your Gastric Bypass" (2004) 1-6

Chapter 12
Dr. Oakley, "Nutritional Guidelines After Your Gastric Bypass" (2004) 2-14

Chapter 15
Definition of Commitment:
American Psychological Association (APA): Commitment. (n.d.). *Dictionary.com Unabridged (v 1.1)*. Retrieved February 28, 2007, from Dictionary.com website: http://dictionary.reference.com/browse/Commitment, "We have made a commitment to pay our bills on time." Changed to: "We have made a commitment to use all the tools of Gastric Bypass Surgery." "They have a sincere commitment to religion." Changed to: "I have a sincere commitment to change my life."

Dr Oakley, Doctor's Corner - Alcohol in Gastric Bypass Patients, (2007) 1-1